Y0-BRA-436

Handbook of Health Assessment

Executive Producer: Rick Weimer
Production Editor: A. Noble
Art Director: Don Sellers

HANDBOOK
of
HEALTH ASSESSMENT

Ellen B. Rudy, R.N., Ph.D.
and
V. Ruth Gray, R.N., M.S.N.

ROBERT J. BRADY CO.
A Prentice-Hall Publishing and Communications
Company
Bowie, Maryland

Handbook of Health Assessment

Copyright © 1981 by Robert J. Brady Co.
All rights reserved. No part of this publication may be reproduced or transmitted in any form or by any means, electronic or mechanical, including photocopying and recording, or by any information storage and retrieval system, without permission in writing from the publisher. For information, address Robert J. Brady Co., Bowie, Maryland 20715.

Library of Congress Cataloging in Publication Data

Rudy, Ellen B
    Handbook of health assessment.
    Includes bibliographical references and index.
    1. Physical diagnosis. 2. Medical history taking.
3. Nursing. I. Gray, V. Ruth, joint author.
II. Title.
RT48.R82   616.07'54   80-24706
ISBN 0-87619-843-4

Prentice-Hall International, Inc., London
Prentice-Hall of Australia, Pty., Ltd., Sydney
Prentice-Hall of India Private Limited, New Delhi
Prentice-Hall of Japan, Inc., Tokyo
Prentice-Hall of Southeast Asia Pte. Ltd., Singapore
Whitehall Books, Limited, Petone, New Zealand

Printed in the United States of America

81 82 83 84 85 86 87 88 89 90   10 9 8 7 6 5 4 3 2 1

CONTENTS

PREFACE

This book is a result of our students' requests for a brief summary of the health history and physical examination, some key physical findings to remember, and an organized format small enough to be carried in a lab coat. No small task! While this book is not intended to replace the excellent textbooks already available on health history, physical examination, and physical diagnosis, it is intended to be a companion book to the major textbooks for the practitioner who is just learning the skills of health history and physical examination, and as a clinical reference for those skilled practitioners who occasionally find themselves in areas outside their medical specialty. This book focuses on the *adult* patient and contains the recording process with special emphasis on the problem oriented record, the components of the health history, physical examination, and selected laboratory data. It is fully expected that some sections will be condensed and others expanded at the discretion and judgment of the practitioner in the clinical setting.

Each section of the physical examination is prefaced by the health history questions relating to a particular body system or organ. This was done to facilitate episodic patient visits when a complete review of systems may not be done. It should be noted that many questions related to body systems and organs overlap. This emphasizes the fact that many signs and symptoms apply to more than one body system.

Anatomical drawings are included in each section of the physical examination, and the steps to be followed in performing the examination. Also included are some of the common and classic physical findings for each organ or body system. Let us emphasize, no book will take the place of good clinical experience in performing health histories and physical examinations. We do feel, however, it will help the beginning practitioner to be more organized, complete and accurate in learning these new skills and serve as a ready reference for the experienced practitioner.

We urge you to *use* the book—write in it, underline it, add new material or information frequently needed. If you make it a part of your clinical equipment, we believe your data base will be more complete and you will improve your clinical practice.

Ellen B. Rudy
V. Ruth Gray

ACKNOWLEDGEMENT

Pascal once said, "Certain authors, when they speak of their work, say 'my book, my commentary' . . . , they would be better to say, 'our book', 'our commentary' . . . since their writings generally contain more of other peoples' good things than their own."

This, then, is our health assessment book. We are indebted to our preceptors who gave unselfishly of their time and knowledge, to our patients for their participation and acceptance, and to the rich substance integrated and synthesized from the vast amount of material already written on this subject. We also acknowledge those who encouraged us from start to finish. We thank our graduate students whose constant requests for this book got us started, our Dean and fellow colleagues in the School of Nursing for their consistent enthusiasm and encouragement, and our individual families whose moral support was necessary for this undertaking.

Ellen B. Rudy
V. Ruth Gray

RECORDING PROCESS

The practitioner will often find it necessary to record patient data utilizing the recording procedure of a particular health care delivery setting. Whatever the procedure or setting, we cannot overemphasize the necessity for a scrupulous, accurate recording of the health history and physical examination. Indeed all important observations and findings, both normal and abnormal, must be recorded. On the other hand, unimportant negative data are of no value and should not clutter the recording. And in those unavoidable situations when complete patient data are not available, a note indicating the specific missing information and the reasons for its absence is necessary.

The Problem Oriented Record (POR) is a tool of the problem oriented system and this system provides a logical, organized, systematic approach to patient care management. It is for this reason that we strongly encourage the adoption and use of the POR. We offer the following information on the POR as an introduction to those who have never used it and as a review to those who have:

The POR is a systematic way of recording patient information.

The POR has four essential components:

(1) *Defined Data Base*
   Subjective information—obtained during the health history including the chief complaint, present illness, past history, patient profile, and review of systems.
   Objective information—obtained from physical

1

examination and laboratory data.

The data base may be comprehensive, obtained from a complete health history and physical examination; or it may be a specific problem, relating only to a presenting illness and important system.

(2) *Complete Problem List*

Emerges after the data base has been collected.

Serves as a table of contents and is the key to all information in the record.

Should contain significant problems, active, potential, and ongoing, which require management over a period of time.

A problem may be a:
Diagnosis, e.g., acute rheumatic fever
Physiologic state, e.g., heart failure
Symptom, e.g., shortness of breath
Sign, e.g., swollen knee
Risk factor, e.g., smokes two packs per day
Sociologic problem, e.g., no hospitalization insurance
Psychiatric psychologic problem, e.g., fear of surgery

(3) *Initial Plans*

Each active, ongoing problem needs a plan of care which includes three parts:
Diagnostic tests—collection of additional data
Therapeutic treatment—medication, e.g., penicillin
Patient and family education

(4) *Progress Notes*

Narrative notes written on SOAP format for each problem:
(S) Subjective data—what the patient tells you
(O) Objective data—physical examination and laboratory data
(A) Assessment—analysis and synthesis of subjective and objective data, e.g., patient is having hematuria

(P) Plan—may be to "continue current plan" or change from the initial plan, e.g., discontinue anticoagulant therapy today.

While the POR initially requires time to record and discipline in thought, it has many advantages:

Can be used by the entire health team.

Provides documentation of comprehensive care.

Prevents oversight of essential information.

Is easily audited.

OUTLINE OF HEALTH HISTORY

Before beginning the actual health history, identifying information should be obtained from the patient or other reliable source. This includes the following:

Name
Address
Phone Number
Social Security Number
Sex
Birth Date
Marital Status
Occupation
Next of Kin

Some points that are helpful in getting a complete and accurate health history include:

Privacy for the interview
Eye contact with the patient
A caring, listening attitude
Listening without bias or being judgmental
Asking the same question in several ways particularly if information is missing or conflicting

I. Chief Complaint and its Duration (CC)

This, in brief, is the answer in the patient's own words to the question, "What brought you here today?". The chief compaint should be in *one* sentence and may include the patient's age, sex, race, occupation, major symptom, and duration.

RELIABILITY. At this point a note should be made as to whether the history was obtained from the patient, relative, friend or physician, the mental condition of the patient and the probable reliability of the history.

II History of Present Illness (P.I.)

This is a well organized, chronological elaboration of the patient's chief complaint from the time of onset until he is seen by you. Describe as accurately as possible the course of the present illness. This history includes:

Duration
Onset
    Date
    Manner (e.g., sudden, gradual)
    Precipitating or predisposing factors

Characteristics and course
    Location
    Quality
    Intensity
    Quantity
    Temporal character
    Aggravating factors
    Relieving factors (including medication)
    Progress

Associated symptoms
Effects of treatment
Past treatment
Past incidence or familial tendency
Ask the patient, "When were you last your normal self?"

The course of the disease should be developed symptomatically in chronological order, each symptom thoroughly developed in its course. When there is a conspicuous disturbance of a particular *organ* or *system,* questions should be asked concerning possible symptoms which refer to the disturbance of this organ or system.

Inquiry should be made concerning any general abnormality and symptoms beyond those already mentioned, e.g., pain, chills, fever, night sweats, weight loss, anorexia, tremors.

Included, finally, is a statement of any continuing problem, i.e., diabetes, obesity, hypertension, heart disease, etc.

III. Past History (P.H.)

GENERAL HEALTH: Statement of health prior to examination.

MEDICAL HISTORY: Previous major illnesses. Diagnosis. Dates. Hospitalized. Complications. Physician.

SURGICAL HISTORY: Procedure. Dates. Complications. Hospital and physician.

OTHER HOSPITALIZATIONS: Diagnosis. Dates. Treatment. Physician. The purpose of this question is to elicit information not covered through medical and surgical past history.

INJURIES AND RESULTING DISABILITIES

ALLERGY: Asthma, hay fever, hives, poison oak, food idiosyncracy, drugs and what kind of reaction. Previous penicillin treatment.

ACUTE INFECTIOUS DISEASES: Acute streptococcal infections, rheumatic fever, infectious mononeucleosis, hepatitis.

If other infections should be mentioned, specific statements must be made concerning them; if there is a history of any acute infections, the duration, severity, complications and sequelae, should be recorded. Inquire about childhood diseases and immunizations for measles, mumps, whooping cough, chicken pox, diptheria, smallpox. Also inquire about unusual reactions to immunizations.

MEDICATIONS: Currently taken and past reactions.

IV. Family History (F.H.)

A family tree diagram is helpful in recording this information. This diagram will indicate the present health of each family member, age, sex, alive or deceased, and incidence of hereditary diseases. Specific inquiry should be made about hereditary and communicable diseases such as diabetes, cystic fibrosis, hemophilia, heart diseases, hypertension, obesity, cancer and tuberculosis. Suggested family tree symbols: ○ = female, □ = male, ● ■ = deceased.

Example: Patient is a 35 year-old male with diabetes mellitus. His mother is 67 years old, living and well; his father died at the age of 52 from heart disease; two sisters, ages 34 and 36 are living and well.

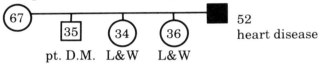

52
heart disease

pt. D.M.   L&W   L&W

V. Socio-cultural History:

Birthplace, education, position in family, marital status, children, residences, military service.

Occupation: exposure to toxins, pollution, physical or mental strain.

Habits: sleep, diet, exercise, alcohol, tobacco, drugs.

Environmental: exposure to contagious disease, hazards, living conditions.

VI. Review of Systems

This part of the history reviews major symptoms as they relate to general body systems. Symptoms revealed may "paint a picture" for clues relating to the patient's present illness. Remember these are *patient* responses and not physical findings.

A SCHEMATIC OF THE PROBLEM-ORIENTED RECORD

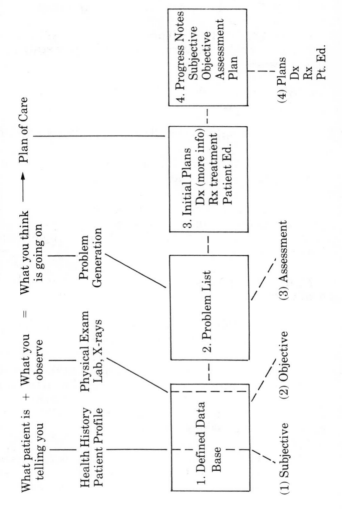

9

SKIN: Rash, eruptions, itching, pigmentation, texture change, moisture, hair growth, bruising, bleeding.

NAILS: Color changes, brittleness, curvature.

HEAD AND SCALP: Headaches, dizziness, syncope, vertigo; hair color, texture, and distribution; scalp itching or lesions.

EYES: Vision, color blindness, diplopia, trauma, inflammatory disease, pain, recent refraction.

EARS: Hearing, earache, discharge, tinnitus, vertigo.

NOSE AND SINUSES: Sense of smell, colds, obstruction, epistaxis, post-nasal drip, sinus pain.

MOUTH AND TEETH: Lesions, soreness, pain, bleeding or receding gums, abscesses, teeth extractions, chewing surfaces, dentures, difficulty chewing or swallowing.

THROAT AND NECK: Sore throats, tonsillitis, hoarseness, neck swelling, stiffness, or pain.

BREASTS: Pain, tenderness, lumps, discharge, changes, breast feeding, gynecomastia.

RESPIRATORY: Pain in chest, dyspnea at rest or with exercise, wheezing, cough, sputum (character and quantity), hemoptysis, night sweats, orthopnea, paroxysmal nocturnal dyspnea, last x-ray of chest and result, including where obtained.

CARDIOVASCULAR: Pain or distress over precordium, radiations of pain, palpitation, changes in rate of rhythm, dyspnea, orthopnea, edema, cyanosis, estimate of exercise tolerance, blood pressure, if known, claudication, varicose veins, phlebitis, last ECG and result, including where obtained.

10

GASTRO-INTESTINAL: Appetite and digestion, change in weight, pain with relation to swallowing or eating, eructation, flatulence, heartburn, nausea, vomiting, hematemesis, regularity of bowels, cathartics, diarrhea, stools (clay colored, tarry, fresh blood), hemorrhoids, hernia, jaundice, dark urine, use of antacids.

GENITO-URINARY: Color, dysuria, pain, passage of gravel, frequency, nocturia, hematuria, polydipsia, polyuria, oliguria, edema of face, hesitancy, dribbling, loss in size and force of stream.

Gonorrhea and Syphilis: Inquire by name (many use street language, i.e., clap). Symptoms, treatment (self or medical), reinfection, present status.

Males: Onset of puberty, voice change, erections, emission, satisfactory sexual adjustment.

Females: Age of menarche, cycle description, dysmenorrhea (primary or secondary), last menstrual period, climacteric symptoms, douching practices, last Pap test, vaginal discharge, medications. Pregnancies, number, problems, complications, infertility problems, type of contraception, dyspareunia, satisfactory sexual adjustment.

MUSCULOSKELETAL: Morning stiffness, backache, pain, joint swelling, muscular weakness or atrophy, cramps.

NEUROLOGICAL: Nervousness, insomnia, drowsiness, vertigo, tremors, convulsions, paralysis, paresthesias, neuralgia, memory, orientation, affect.

LYMPHATIC: Swollen lymph nodes, pain.

HEMATOPOIETIC: Anemia, tendency to bruise or bleed, thrombosis, thrombophlebitis, blood transfusions and reactions.

ENDOCRINE: Relative size of body including back, feet and head, hair distribution and texture, enlargement of thyroid, intolerance to heat or cold, weakness, exophthalmia, tremor, polyphagia, polydipsia, polyuria, glycosuria.

Ask the patient these general questions at the end of the history:
"Is there anything else that concerns you?"
"What problem concerns you the most?"

─────────────┤**3**├─────────────

INTRODUCTION TO ROUTINE PHYSICAL EXAMINATION

Before beginning the outline of the portions of the physical examination, several points should be emphasized. The organization of the physical examination is not based on the body system approach characteristic of the study of physiology. Instead, the patient is examined in a *series of steps* starting at the head and generally moving down the body. The approach is intended to gather as much information as possible on function, size, and appearance of organs and body parts to make a comprehensive and integrated evaluation of the presence or absence of pathology and the total body response to pathological processes.

A complete health history should be done before any part of the physical examination is performed. The exceptions are, of course, emergency situations or when the patient exhibits extreme pain, shortness of breath or other symptoms making a health history impossible. The major purpose of a good health history is to give the examiner clues as to physical problems which should be explored and verified in the physical examination. There are aspects of the patient's illness which are revealed only by physical examination. For these reasons, it is important that the physical examination be done thoroughly, skillfully, and in a logical sequence.

The four classical techniques of the physical examination are:

Inspection
Palpation
Percussion
Auscultation

These will be utilized when appropriate during each portion of the physical examination.

Record: Temperature
          Pulse
          Respirations
          Blood pressure (note position of patient and
              limb used)
          Height
          Weight

A general introduction to the physical examination should provide a picture of the "patient-as-a-whole." It includes the patient's mental status, body development, nutritional state, chronological versus apparent age, presenting appearance and speech. It also includes the character of the patient's general condition—presence of pain, shortness of breath, restlessness, tremors, coma.

|4|

SKIN

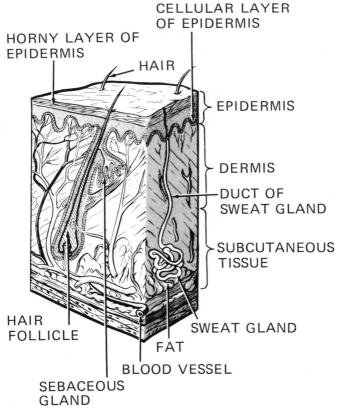

CELLULAR LAYER
OF EPIDERMIS

HORNY LAYER OF
EPIDERMIS

HAIR

EPIDERMIS

DERMIS

DUCT OF
SWEAT GLAND

SUBCUTANEOUS
TISSUE

HAIR
FOLLICLE

SWEAT GLAND

FAT

BLOOD VESSEL

SEBACEOUS
GLAND

Figure 4-1. Anatomy of the Skin

15

History Questions

Rash
  Description, location, onset
  Accompanying symptoms as itching, pain
  Allergies
Exposure to contagious skin conditions
Lesions
  Descriptions, location, onset
  Accompanying symptoms as itching, pain
Recent color changes
  Vitiligo, hyperpigmentation, jaundice
Change in moles
  Color, shape, size, sensitivity, itching
Vascular changes
  Petechiae, ecchymosis, bruising, spider angioma
Psychological response
  Withdrawal from social activities
  Cosmetics
  Change in self-image

Examination

The techniques of inspection and palpation are used principally in examination of the skin. The fingertips are sensitive to fine tactile detail and are therefore best suited to palpating lesions and masses; the thin dorsal aspects of the fingers or hands are best suited to palpating skin temperature.

Inspection and Palpation. Inspect and palpate general overall and specific skin areas beginning with hands, forearms and face and continuing throughout the physical examination.
  Note:
    Color: Pallor, flushing, cyanosis, redness, brownness, jaundice
    Vascularity: Dilated superficial veins, evidence of bleeding or bruising, petechiae, ecchymosis
    Temperature: Feel skin to assess increased local warmth or coolness

Texture: Roughness, smoothness, thickness
Moisture: Dryness, sweating, oiliness
Mobility and turgor: Ease with which the skin
  moves (mobility) and returns to place (turgor)

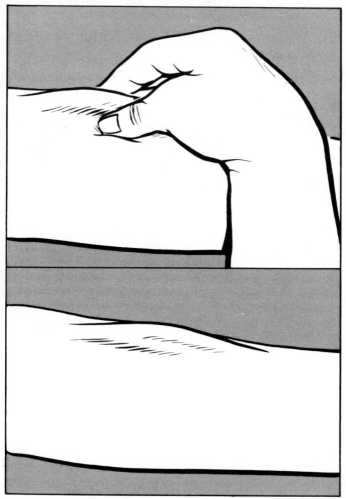

Figure 4-2. Testing for skin turgor

In dehydration, senile cutaneous atrophy, or rapid loss of body tissue, skin turgor is diminished. Loss of turgor is evident when the skin remains in a fold after pinching. This is referred to as "tenting."

Lesions should be described in the following manner:

Color

Size

Configuration (diffuse, discrete, well circumscribed)

Shape consistency (soft, hard)

Odor

Effect of pressure

Pulsatility

Distribution over body—localized or generalized—on exposed skin surface or skin folds

Arrangement (clustered, linear, annular)

Relationship to hair follicle

Primary and/or secondary lesions

Primary lesions develop without any preceding skin changes.

Secondary lesions result from changes in primary lesions and are influenced by scratching, infection, and treatment.

Table 4-1. Primary Lesions

Lesion	Description	Example	Figure
Macule	Change in skin color Less than 1 cm. No change in consistency or elevation of skin Can be caused by inflammatory dilation of small blood vessels Not palpable	Freckles Flat moles Rubella Drug eruptions First degree burns Lupus erythematosus	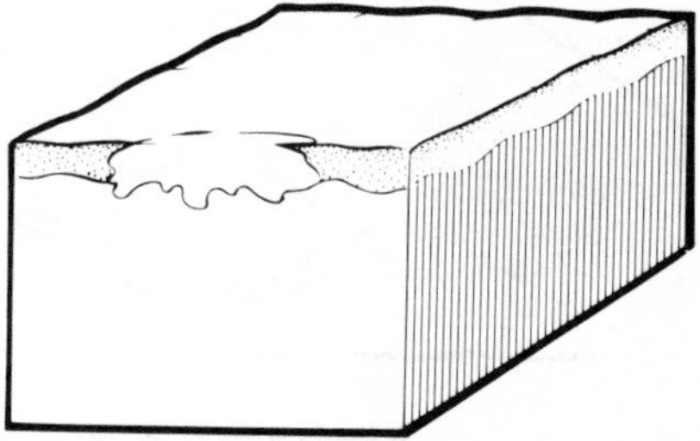
Papule	Circumscribed *solid* elevation Not over 1 cm.	Lichen Planus Some warts Acne Insect bites Psoriasis	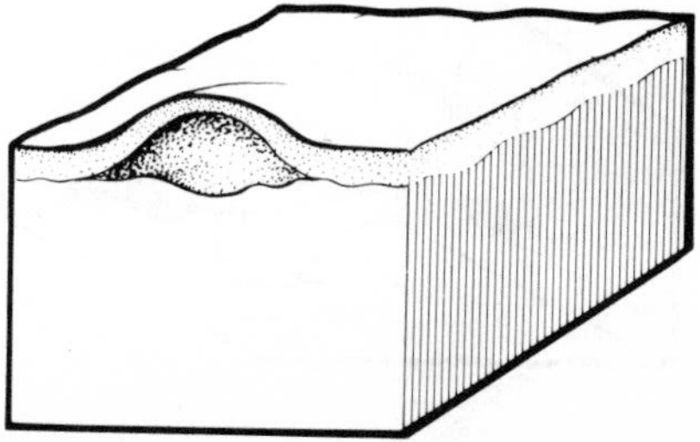

19

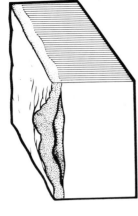

Nodule

Increased elevation or consistency over papule
1-2 cm.
Can be soft or hard

Nodulus Cutaneous
Pigmented nevi
Gummas
Xanthomas

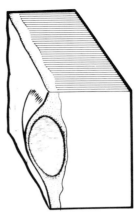

Tumor

Solid mass
Over 2 cm.

Dermatofibroma
Epithelioma

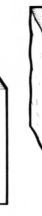
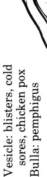
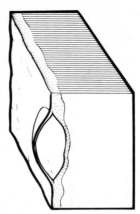

Wheal

Fluid held diffusely in tissue, temporarily raising skin (contains no blood or free fluid)

1 mm. to several cm.

Urticaria
Mosquito bites

Vesicle or *Bulla*

Circumscribed elevation

Serous fluid flows easily if wall is punctured

Vesicle: less than 1 cm.;
Bulla: more than 1 cm.

Vesicle: blisters, cold sores, chicken pox
Bulla: pemphigus

21

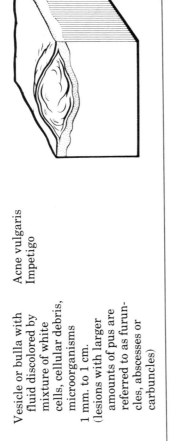

Pustule

Vesicle or bulla with fluid discolored by mixture of white cells, cellular debris, microorganisms 1 mm. to 1 cm. (lesions with larger amounts of pus are referred to as furuncles, abscesses or carbuncles)

Acne vulgaris
Impetigo

Table 4-2. Secondary Lesions

Lesions	Description	Example	Figure
Crust	Thickened, dried-out fluid From serous fluid, purulent infection or blood oozing	Impetigo Eczema	
Plaque	Lesion resulting from coalescence of wheals Large elevated plateau-like lesion	Hives	

23

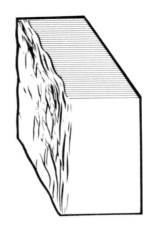

Pustule   Infected papule (may   Acne
also be primary)

Scale   Excess of horny mater-   Pityriasis rosea
ial on skin's surface   Psoriasis
Flakes of skin

24

Fissure

Linear break in
epidermis
Crack in skin surface
Erosion (scoop out
break in epidermis;
no scarring)

Eczema
Chapping

Ulcer

Deeper break in
epidermis; may ex-
tend deeply into
corium and sub-
cutaneous tissue;
may scar.

Chancre
Stasis ulcer

25

Scar

Skin repaired with fibrous tissue or excess collagen

Postoperative scar
Keloid

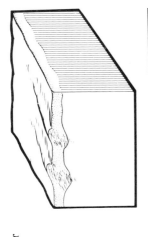

Skin conditions in persons with dark skin may be difficult to assess. Examine dark skin utilizing the following considerations.

Table 4-3. Skin Conditions

Condition	Consideration
Petechiae	Usually appear in mucous membranes in diseases manifesting petechiae Inspect buccal mucosa and the bulbar and palpebral conjunctiva

Erythema	Associated with rash, palpate for papular type lesion From carbon monoxide poisoning and polycythemias, observe lips.
Ecchymosis	Differentiate from erythema, pressure on skin causes erythema to blanch Inspect buccal mucosa and the conjunctivae
Pallor (absence of un- derlying red tones which give dark skin a glow)	Will appear yellowish brown or ashen gray Inspect mucosa membrane, lips and nail beds
Cyanosis	Need to be familiar with person's precyanotic state Inspect lips, nails, ear lobes, palpebral conjunctiva Apply pressure on tissue, color returns normally in less than one second. In cyanosis, color returns by spreading more slowly from periphery to center of area where pressure applied.
Jaundice	Inspect sclera when eye lids are in regular visual position. Can be confused with pigmentation (some persons normally have subconjunctival fat with carotene which becomes darker further from cornea). If yellowish near cornea, jaundice may be present.

Inspection and Palpation. Inspect and palpate the fingernails and toenails noting color, shape, lesions, general condition.

Table 4-4. Abnormalities or Variations of Nails

Abnormality or Variation	Cause	Figure
Badly mutilated, bitten	Usually nervous habit of biting	
Beau's line	Matrix forms transverse indentation during severe illness	

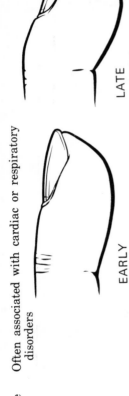

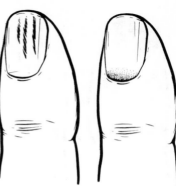

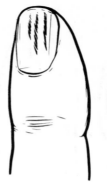

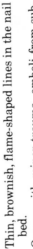

EARLY

LATE

Clubbing: Early, Late

Often associated with cardiac or respiratory disorders

Splinter hemorrhages

Thin, brownish, flame-shaped lines in the nail bed.
Occurs with minor trauma, emboli from sub-acute bacterial endocarditis or without specific cause

Red half-moons in nail bed

Cardiac failure

29

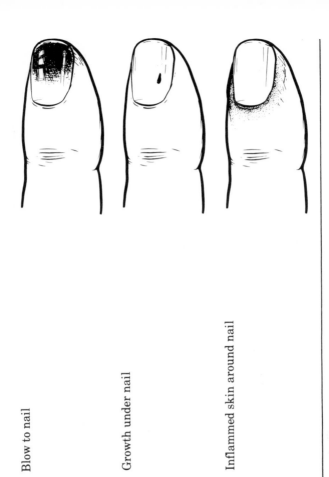

Subungual hematoma   Blow to nail

Subungual glomus tumor   Growth under nail

Paronychia   Inflammed skin around nail

5

HEAD AND NECK

The Head

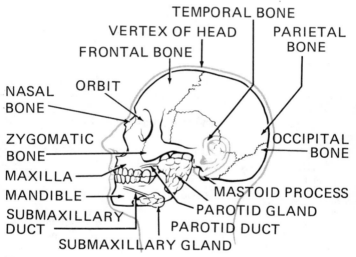

Figure 5-1. Lateral View of Skull

History Questions

Headache
 Quality, location, severity, visual disturbance, nausea, vomiting, syncope, vertigo
 Radiation to neck and shoulders
 Migraine
 Provocative or palliative factors, i.e., position of head
 History of hypertension
 Medication
Past injuries
 Severity, treatment, residual
Any noticeable changes
 Hair texture and amount
 Facial sensation, symmetry
 Facial skin texture and moisture

Examination

Inspection and Palpation. Inspect and palpate:
Hair
 If wig is worn, remove for hair and skull examination
 Quality, distribution, texture, pattern of loss
 Differentiate between nits and dandruff
Scalp
 Hygiene, lumps, lesions
Skull
 General size and contour, deformities, depressions, lumps, or presence of underlying tenderness
Skin
 Color, pigmentation, texture, lesion, hair distribution
Face
 Facial expression and symmetry, areas of anesthesia or differences in touch sensation

Table 5-1   Skull Characteristics that May be Signs of Particular Conditions

Characteristic	Condition
Abnormally small head	Associated with mental retardation
Abnormally large head	Associated with hydrocephalus or acromegaly
Abnormally elongated skull	Sometimes seen in sickle cell anemia

Table 5-2   Hair Characteristics that May be Signs of Particular Conditions

Characteristics	Condition
Dryness, brittleness	Myxedema, aging
Fine, silky	Hyperthyroidism
Alopecia	Secondary syphilis Severe emotional stress Cytotoxic drugs for treatment of malignancy
Smooth, round lesions, attached to overlying skin	Sebaceous cyst or wen
Crusts and flakes	Eczema, seborrheic dermatitis, dandruff, psoriasis Contact dermatitis from hair dye or spray

Expression	Condition
Grotesque, grinning expression due to spasm of facial muscles	Tetanus
Flat, expressionless, masklike faces with occasional drooling	Paralysis agitans (Parkinsonism)
Velvety smooth skin, wide-eyed, startled expression	Hyperthyroidism (with exophthalmus)
Faintly confused or quizzical expression	Deafness
Perpetual frown or squint	Poor vision
Expression of exhaustion or defeat	Malignant and chronic wasting disease
Asymmetry of facial structures	Paresis or paralysis of facial muscles
Elevations of the skin surface over the nose, lips, cheeks, forehead or temple	Lipomas and basal cell or squamous cell carcinoma
Coarse, thickened facial skin which may produce a dull, sleepy expression, orbital edema	Hypothyroidism

The Neck

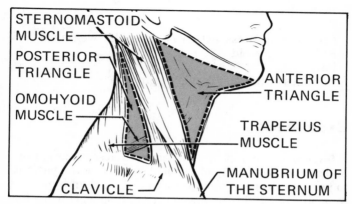

Figure 5-2. Anatomy of Neck Muscles

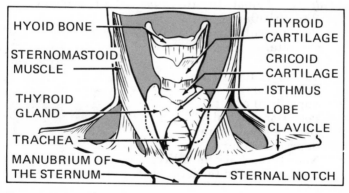

Figure 5-3. Internal Anatomy of Neck

35

History Questions

    Lumps in neck, hoarseness, swelling
    Difficulty swallowing
    Swollen glands
    Frequent stiffness, arthritis, muscular weakness
    Enlarged thyroid
    Pain
    Changes of ROM of cervical spine

Examination

Inspection. Inspect for symmetry, masses, scars, normal cervical concavity of cervical spine. Ask the patient to perform range of motion including flexion, hyperextension, lateral flexion and rotation. Inspect trachea for any deviation from midline and difficulty swallowing and for venous jugular distention.

Palpation. Palpate the 10 *lymph nodes* in sequence.
    Pre-auricular
    Post-auricular
    Occipital
    Parotid
    Submaxillary
    Submental
    Superficial cervical
    Posterior cervical
    Deep cervical chain
    Supraclavicular
    Note: Size, shape, mobility,
    consistency and tenderness of
    nodes.
Palpate *trachea* to determine proper alignment.

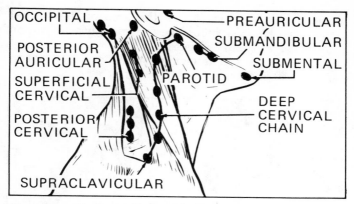

Figure 5-4. The Lymph Nodes of the Head and Neck

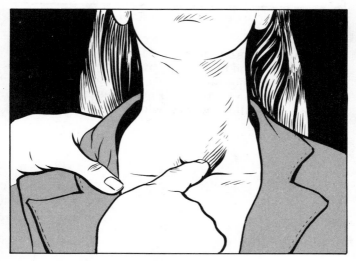

Figure 5-5. Palpation of the Trachea

37

Place finger over trachea in the area of the sternal notch. The trachea should be far enough posterior to allow a finger tip to be inserted.

Palpate *thyroid* to determine size, shape, symmetry, tenderness, nodules.

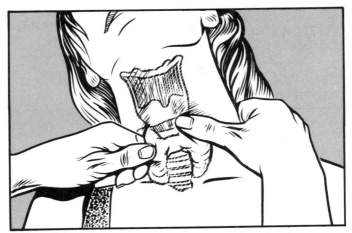

Figure 5-6a. Palpation of Thyroid from Front

Rest your thumbs on the nape of the patient's neck and with the index and middle fingers of both hands feel for the thyroid isthmus and for the anterior surfaces of the lateral lobes. The thyroid will move past the fingertip (upward) on swallowing. See below

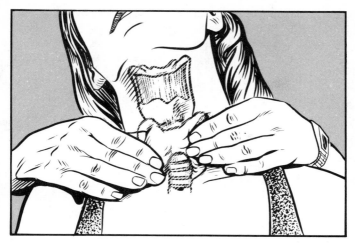

Figure 5-6b. Palpation of Thyroid from Behind

Palpate *carotid arteries* and *jugular veins*. Note rhythm, volume, equality of sides. Palpate only one side at a time to avoid carotid sinus massage.

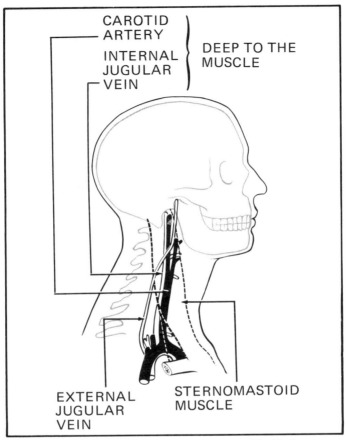

Figure 5-7. Jugular Veins and Carotid Artery of the Neck

Auscultation. Auscultate carotid pulses for rhythm, volume, weakness, bruits, or radiation of murmurs.

6

MOUTH AND PHARYNX

History Questions

Lesions or soreness of mouth or tongue
  Onset, cause, treatment
Difficulty with gums
  Bleeding, recession, bismuth lines, pain
Change in color of lips
Previous surgery
  Gums, mouth
Voice changes
  Onset, duration, treatment
Difficulty swallowing
Sore throat
  Frequency, treatment

Examination

Inspection. Inspect the mouth and throat in the following order:
  Lips for color, moisture, lumps, ulcer, cracking, ulcerative lesions, symmetry.
  Buccal mucosa and parotid duct orifice for color, pigmentation, ulcer, nodules.
  Gums for inflammation, swelling, bleeding, retraction, hypertrophy or discoloration.
  Teeth for looseness, caries, partial plate, abnormal position, biting, chewing surface.

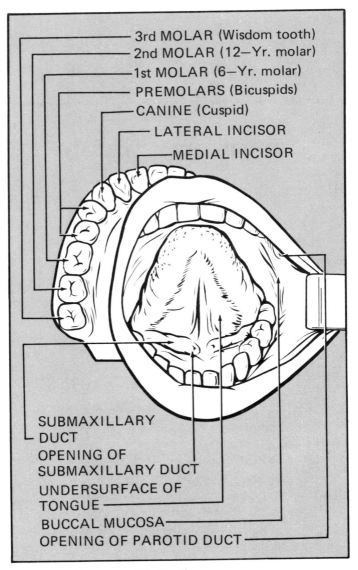

3rd MOLAR (Wisdom tooth)
2nd MOLAR (12—Yr. molar)
1st MOLAR (6—Yr. molar)
PREMOLARS (Bicuspids)
CANINE (Cuspid)
LATERAL INCISOR
MEDIAL INCISOR

SUBMAXILLARY
DUCT
OPENING OF
SUBMAXILLARY DUCT
UNDERSURFACE OF
TONGUE
BUCCAL MUCOSA
OPENING OF PAROTID DUCT

Figure 6-1. Structures of the Mouth

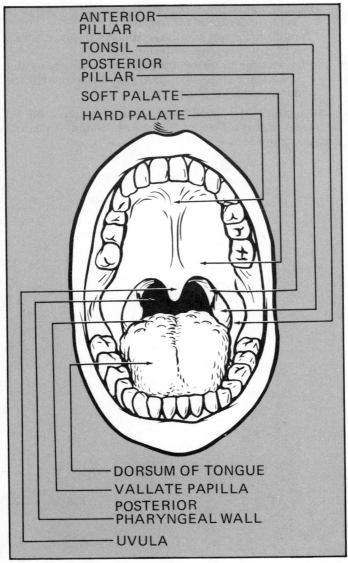

ANTERIOR PILLAR

TONSIL

POSTERIOR PILLAR

SOFT PALATE

HARD PALATE

DORSUM OF TONGUE

VALLATE PAPILLA

POSTERIOR PHARYNGEAL WALL

UVULA

Figure 6-2. The Mouth and the Pharynx

43

Roof of mouth for color, architecture of hard palate (remove dentures for inspection).

Tongue for color, papillae, abnormal smoothness, mid-line, presence of lesions.

Pharynx for anterior and posterior pillars, uvula; tonsils for color, symmetry, enlargement, exudate; posterior pharynx.

Palpation. With gloved hand, palpate lesion of the lip or buccal mucosa, floor of the mouth, tongue to detect masses or tenderness.

────────────| 7 |────────────

NOSE AND SINUSES

History Questions

Nasal discharge
 Known allergies, epistaxis
Ability to smell
 Stuffiness, polyps
Frequent colds
 Allergic rhinitis, post nasal drip
 Medication
Related surgery
 T & A, deviated septum
Frequent headaches

Examination

Inspection. Inspect nose for deformity, asymmetry, inflammation.

Nasal mucosa for color, moisture, swelling, bleeding, exudate of mucosa.
Nasal septum for deviation, perforation, bleeding.
Inferior turbinates and possibly middle turbinates for color, moisture, exudate, polyps.

Palpation. Palpate frontal sinuses and maxillary for soreness or tenderness. Transilluminate sinuses

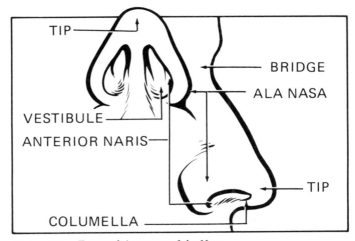

Figure 7-1. External Anatomy of the Nose

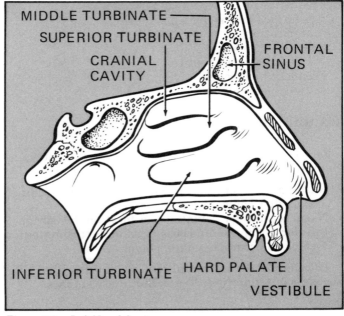

Figure 7-2. Left Nasal Cavity

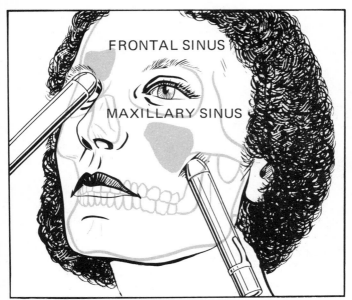

Figure 7-3. Transillumination of Sinus Cavities

8

EYE

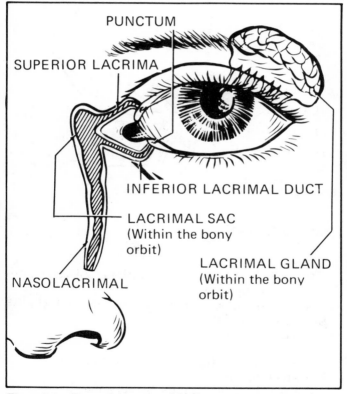

Figure 8-1. External Anatomy of the Eye

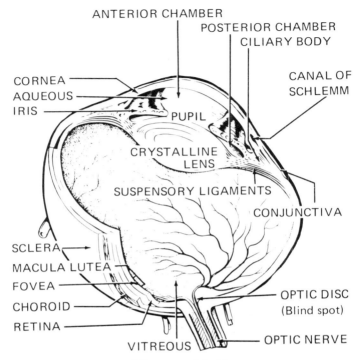

ANTERIOR CHAMBER

POSTERIOR CHAMBER
CILIARY BODY

CORNEA
AQUEOUS
IRIS

CANAL OF
SCHLEMM

PUPIL

CRYSTALLINE
LENS

SUSPENSORY LIGAMENTS

CONJUNCTIVA

SCLERA
MACULA LUTEA
FOVEA
CHOROID
RETINA

OPTIC DISC
(Blind spot)

VITREOUS

OPTIC NERVE

Figure 8-2. Anatomical Structure of the Eye

History Questions

Difficulty with vision
  Blurring with near objects, with far objects, photo-
    phobia, diplopia
  Night blindness, color blindness, halo around lights
Evidence of eye fatigue
  Tiredness, headaches
Inflammation
  Hyperemia, itching, burning, tearing, pain
Known problems
  Cornea, iris, nystagmus, strabismus, hordeolum,
    chalazion

Examination

Perform tests for:

Visual Acuity

Snellen chart for distance vision

Pocket card or news print for near vision

Visual Fields

Gross confrontation of the visual fields is tested by comparing the patient's peripheral vision with the examiner's vision (assuming normal vision of examiner). With examiner and patient facing each other, one eye is covered and the examiner brings a wiggling finger into the visual fields until it is seen by the patient. This is repeated for each visual field and for each eye. Note any visual field deficits.

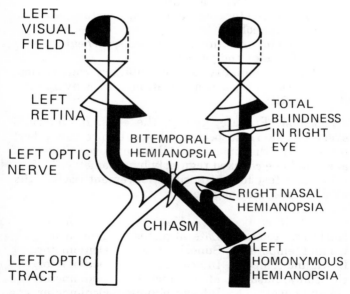

Figure 8-3. Schematic Drawing of Visual Fields: Including Visual Field Defects

Corneal Light Reflex
Determine symmetrical or asymmetrical position of light reflections on the right and left eyes.

External Eye
Inspection. Inspect the eye, its orbit and surrounding tissue.

Eyebrows for distribution, position, alignment, and movement
Eyelashes for distribution, color, texture, and position
Eyelids for color, edema, mobility, superficial vascularity, position-alignment
Lacrimal apparatus for swelling, tenderness and redness
Orbit for forward or backward displacement of the eye in its socket and alignment
Conjunctiva for color, injection, moisture, lesions
Sclera for color
Cornea for smoothness, clearness, corneal reflex
Iris for color and pattern
Pupil for equality, shape, pupillary constriction, consensual, accommodation and convergence, PERRLA

Palpation. Palpate, gently, the eyes. If abnormal eyeball tension is suspected, intraocular pressure is best measured by the tonometer. All persons over 40 years of age should be checked regularly by tonometry.

Perform test for extraocular movement (EOM). Six cardinal positions of gaze.

Position	Muscle	Nerve
Horizontal temporal	Lateral rectus	Trochlear
Up and temporal	Superior rectus	Oculomotor
Down and temporal	Inferior rectus	Oculomotor
Horizontal nasal	Medial rectus	Oculomotor
Up and nasal	Inferior oblique	Oculomotor
Down and nasal	Superior oblique	Abducens

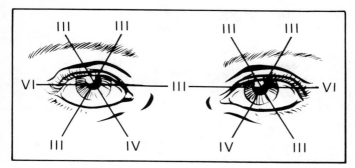

Figure 8-4. Cardinal Positions of Gaze

Internal Eye
Inspection. (Fundoscopy) The procedure for ophthalmoscopy requires the following considerations.

Your right hand and right eye are used to examine the patient's right eye; the left hand and eye for the patient's left eye. The room should be darkened; the ophthalmoscope set at 0 diopters. Position your thumb on the patient's eyebrow. Ask patient to look straight ahead and fix his gaze on a specific point on the wall.

Hold ophthalmoscope against your face, center your eye behind the sight hole. Your index finger will be on the lens disc of the ophthalmoscope.

While standing 15 inches from the patient and about 15° lateral to his line of vision, shine the light beam on his pupil.

As you follow the light beam through the patient's pupil, adjust the lens disc of the opthalmoscope to facilitate visualization of the internal structure of the eye.

Inspect the following:

> Red reflex
> Lens for clearness and transparency
> Optic disc for size, shape, color, physiologic cup depression normal (disc/cup ratio .2/1.0) and margins
> Blood vessels for pathways, contours, A/V ratio, venous pulsations, A/V crossings and light reflexes
> Macula and Fovea Centralis

53

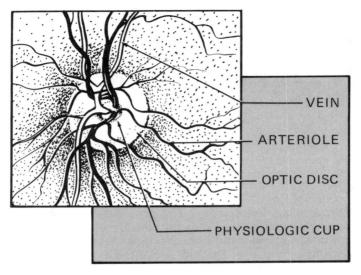

Figure 8-5. Optic Disc and Blood Vessels

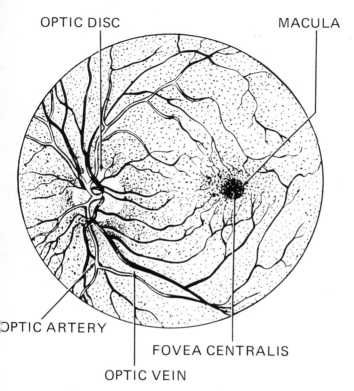

OPTIC DISC MACULA

OPTIC ARTERY FOVEA CENTRALIS

OPTIC VEIN

Figure 8-6. Fundus of the Eye

Table 8-1. Some Abnormalities on Ophthalmoscopy

Finding	Interpretation	Example
Pale white disc; pallor extends to disc margins; disc vessels absent	Death of optic nerve fibers	Optic atrophy
Disc margins blurred; physiologic cup not visible, disc appears to project forward (Papilledema)	Venous stasis	Increased intracranial pressure Mass lesions Hypertension
Base of cup pale; cup enlarged and extends to edge of disc	Increased intraocular pressure	Glaucoma
Arteries change color, become opaque, show copper wire or silver wire defect	Thickening of the retinal arteriole	Aging Arteriosclerosis Hypertension
Tiny red spots commonly located in the macular area	Microaneurysms	Diabetic retinopathy

Vein stops abruptly or tapers on either side of arteriole	Arteriovenous nicking	Aging Arteriosclerosis With or without hypertension Retinal diseases
Streaked flame-shaped hemorrhages paralleling the blood vessels	Capillary insufficiency or ischemia	Hypertensive retinopathy
Fluffy, white "soft" exudate (cotton wool patches)	Hypertensive changes of a terminal arteriole; thickening and swelling of the terminal retinal nerve fibers.	Diabetes Connective tissue disease Hypertension Papilledema
Round, yellowish-white deposits in retina (hard exudate)	Edema residues from leaking capillaries or arterioles or degenerating nerve tissue	Hypertension Diabetes

9

EAR

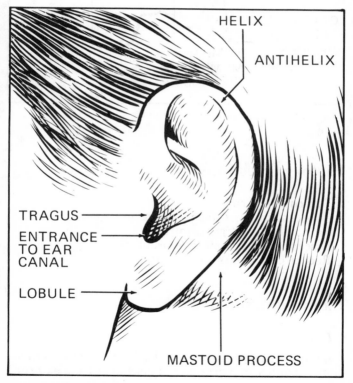

Figure 9-1. External Anatomy of the Ear

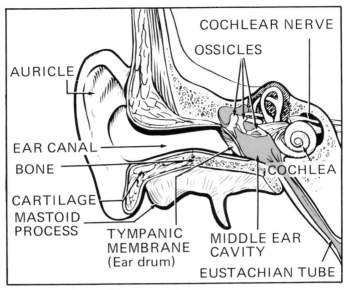

Figure 9-2. Internal Anatomy of the Ear

History Questions

Difficulty hearing
  Recent changes, factor affecting this
Pain in ear, vertigo, tinnitus
Discharge, past history of problems
Recent URI, allergies, sinusitis

Examination

External Ear

Inspection. Inspect both auricles for color, size, skin lesions, nodules, and presence of discharge from external canal.

60

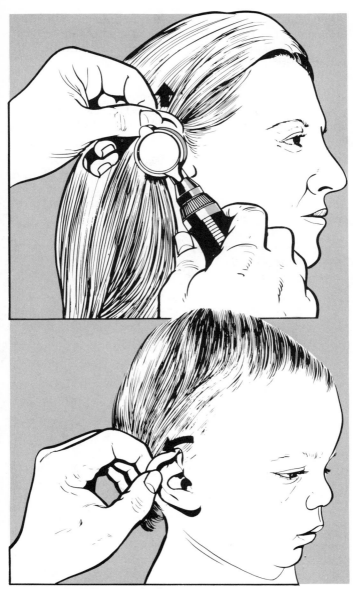

Figure 9.3. Ear Position for Otoscopy

61

Palpation. Palpate auricles for nodules, tophi, and tenderness by pulling on pinna and pushing on tragus. *Note.* Movements of pinna and tragus are painful with external otitis, but not with otitis media.

Internal Ear

Inspection. Pull auricle upward and backward in adult and downward and back in child to straighten auditory canal and insert otoscope.

Examine auditory canal as otoscope is inserted.

Identify wax (cerumen), discharge, tumors or foreign bodies in ear canal. Identify tympanic membrane (TM) and landmarks—malleus (manubrium and short process), umbo, cone of light, and annulus.

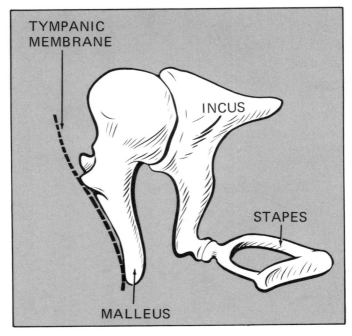

TYMPANIC MEMBRANE

INCUS

STAPES

MALLEUS

Figure 9.4. Bones of the Ear

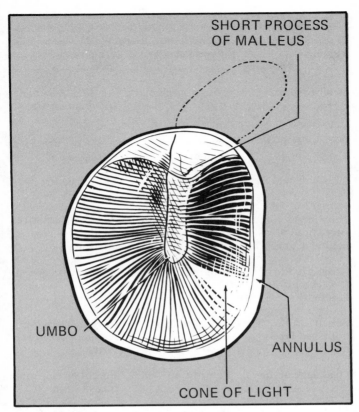

SHORT PROCESS OF MALLEUS

UMBO

ANNULUS

CONE OF LIGHT

Figure 9.5. Landmarks of the Tympanic Membrane

Move speculum to see entire drum. Note color and luster of TM, position of malleus and any lesions or abnormalities of TM.

Function–Hearing Test. There are several hearing tests which can be used to get a rough estimate of the patient's hearing acuity. All of these are merely screening tests, and if a hearing loss is identified, a more sophisticated audiometer examination is necessary to determine the degree and range of hearing loss that is present.

Table 9-1   Some Abnormalities on Otoscopy

Finding	Interpretation	Examples
Bright red drum	Inflammation	Acute middle ear infection (otitis media)
Yellowish drum	Pus or serum behind drum	Acute or chronic otitis media
Bluish drum	Blood behind drum	Skull fracture
Hairline meniscus curve or bubbles behind drum	Serous fluid in middle ear	Acute serous otitis media or chronic otitis media
Absent light reflex, obscure landmarks	Bulging of drum	Acute otitis media
Absent or diminished landmarks	Thickening of drum	Chronic otitis media or otitis externa
Oval dark areas	Perforation	Recent or old rupture of drum
Malleus very prominent	Retraction of drum	Obstruction of Eustachian tube

From Sherman J, and Fields S: *Guide to Patient Evaluation.* Medical Examination Publishing Co., Inc., New York, 1978. Used with permission of the publisher.

Watch ticking/whispered voice. Estimate the distance from each ear at which the patient can hear the ticking and compare to person (examiner if possible) with normal hearing. Have patient occlude one ear at a time and, after making sure patient cannot read your lips, whisper clearly a phrase or several words until patient can repeat the words. Repeat procedure with both ears noting differences in perception between ears and level of voice needed for patient to hear (i.e., soft whisper, loud whisper, normal voice, loud voice).

Weber test. Strike tuning fork and holding it by its stem, press firmly against skull in midline. Ask patient in which ear sound is heard best. Should be heard equally well in both ears. A definite *lateralization* to one ear is abnormal.

Rinné test. Strike tuning fork and place stem on mastoid process until patient can no longer hear the sound. Then quickly place tuning fork near ear canal and check if sound can be heard. Normally, air conduction is better than bone conduction (AC>BC). Repeat with other ear and record findings.

Hearing loss is divided into two major areas, conduction loss and sensorineural or perceptive hearing loss. The Weber and Rinné test can help distinguish between these two.

	Weber Test	**Rinné Test**
Conduction loss	Lateralized to *poor* ear because poor ear is not distracted by room noise, sound perceived better in this ear.	BC>AC Normal conduction through ear blocked and bone vibrations bypass blockage.
Sensorineural Loss (nerve loss)	Lateralizes to *good* ear, nerve loss in poor ear unable to receive vibrations.	AC>BC Normal pattern even in poor ear as nerve loss unable to receive vibrations by either route.

Function—Vestibular

Romberg. Have patient stand with feet together and eyes open. If he does not begin to fall, have the patient close his eyes. With labyrinthine stimulation, the patient tends to fall in the direction of the flow of endolymph. Falling may also indicate neurological impairment. Be prepared to catch the patient when test is performed!

|10|

BREAST AND AXILLA

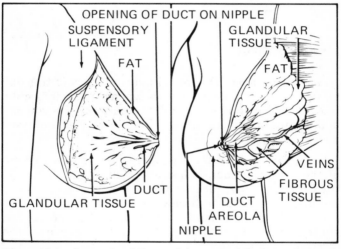

Figure 10-1. Internal and External Anatomy of the Breast

History Questions

Self-examination
  When in menstrual cycle
  How often
Lumps or masses in breast
  Past history and disposition
  Present condition, description, first noticed, how
  discovered

Pain or tenderness in breast
  Description
  Relationship to menses
Discharge from nipples
  Description, onset
  Relationship to menses
Change in size of breast
  Relationship to menses
  Pregnancy or lactation
Pain in axilla
  Enlarged lymph nodes
  Rash or lesions

Examination

Patient education. The most important part of this examination for female patients is teaching or reinforcing routine self-examination. Ask the patient, "Do you examine your breasts regularly? Please show me how you do it?"

Inspection. Inspect for size, shape, symmetry (asymmetry not uncommon unless a *new* finding), nipple retraction, dimpling, "orange peel" skin, venous pattern, lesions, ulcerations or discharge.

Have the patient perform the following maneuvers while in a sitting position and carefully observe for retractions or dimpling:

Raise hands above head
Clasp hands together in front of waist and push arms together forcefully to contract chest muscles.

Inspect axilla and supraclavicular area for retractions, edema or lesion.

Palpation. If patient has noted lump in breast, have her point it out, then palpate *opposite* breast first.

Palpate nipples and areolar area first to determine tenderness, nodules or discharge.

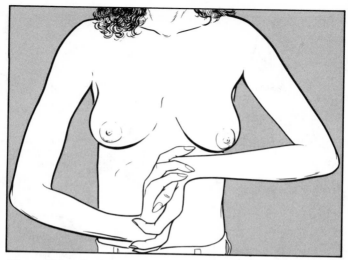

Figure 10-2. Contraction of Pectoral Muscles for Breast Exam

Put patient supine with small pillow under scapula. Carefully palpate entire area of breast in an overlapping fashion being careful not to neglect tail of breast which extends toward axilla. Pattern for palpation may be either quadrants or concentric circles; just make sure *all breast tissue is palpated.*

Palpate axillae, supra and infraclavicular area for lymph nodes.

Masses should be described in the following manner:

Location (quadrant of breast; a sketch of location is helpful)

Size

Contour

Consistency

Mobility

Tenderness or pain

Other features (pulsation, color, accompanying features)

69

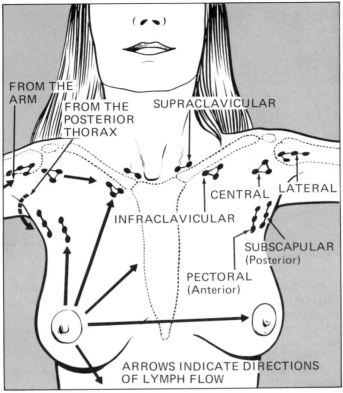

FROM THE ARM
FROM THE POSTERIOR THORAX
SUPRACLAVICULAR
CENTRAL
LATERAL
INFRACLAVICULAR
SUBSCAPULAR (Posterior)
PECTORAL (Anterior)
ARROWS INDICATE DIRECTIONS OF LYMPH FLOW

Figure 10-3. Lymph Glands of the Breast

Special emphasis on self-breast examination should be given to women in high risk groups for breast cancer. These include:

Advanced age

Previous personal history of breast cancer

History of breast cancer in a mother or a sister

History of breast cancer in a maternal or paternal grandmother, father's sister, or mother's sister

History of nodular fibrocystic breasts

Birth of first baby after age of 30

Nulliparity (never borne children)

Early menarche and late menopause

Excessive exposure to ionizing radiation

History of cancer of the endometrium, ovary or colon

Large body size (particularly related to obesity and/or high intake of animal fats)

Estrogen replacement therapy (DHEW Pub. No. 79-1691, 1979)

THORAX AND LUNGS

History Questions

Cough
  How long, productive, increasing frequency
Sputum
  Description and amount
Hemoptysis
  When, amount, frequency, description
Wheezing
  Onset, asthma, allergies, medications
Shortness of breath
  When you first noticed it
  When it bothers you most
  How far can walk or exercise, number of stairs
  How relieved
  Medications
Difficulty breathing at night
  Number of pillows to sleep, recent change
Pain in chest
  Description, onset, radiation, relief, medication

Examination

Inspection. Inspect thorax for size, shape, contour and movement of chest.

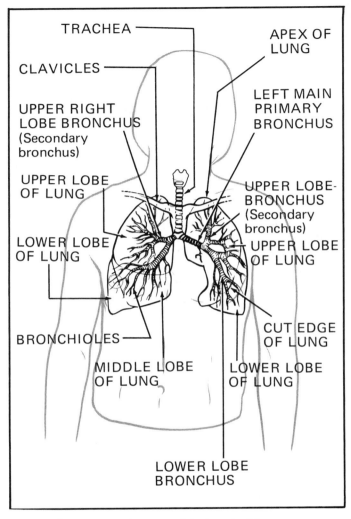

Figure 11-1. Anatomy of the Anterior Thorax

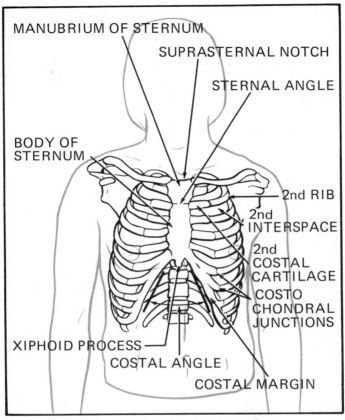

MANUBRIUM OF STERNUM

SUPRASTERNAL NOTCH

STERNAL ANGLE

BODY OF STERNUM

2nd RIB

2nd INTERSPACE

2nd COSTAL CARTILAGE

COSTO CHONDRAL JUNCTIONS

XIPHOID PROCESS

COSTAL ANGLE

COSTAL MARGIN

Figure 11-2. Anatomy of the Respiratory System

Table 11-1   Chest Deformities

Chest Deformity	Description	Sketch
Barrel chest	*Increase in A-P diameter, sternum appears pulled forward, ribs more horizontal*	

Pigeon breast or chicken breast

A-P diameter increased with transverse diameter narrowed vertical grooves in line of costochondral junction

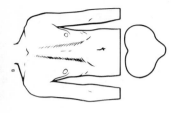

Pectus Excavatum or funnel chest

Ribs of lower part of sternum sink posteriorly creating a pit (excavatum or funnel), this decreases the A-P diameter

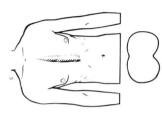

Table 11-2 Spinal Deformities

Spinal Deformities	Description	Sketch
Scoliosis (A)	Lateral curvature of the spine	
Kyphosis (B)	Increase in normal curvature of spine (hump back)	
Lordosis (C)	Concave curvature of spine	

Observe respiratory pattern for puffed cheeks, use of axillary muscles, muscle retraction or abnormal patterns such as:

Cheyne-Stokes Respirations
An irregular or cyclic pattern of breathing characterized by periods of apnea lasting 10-20 seconds.

Kussmaul Respiration
Characterized by deep, regular, sigh-like respirations. Rate may be fast, normal or slow.

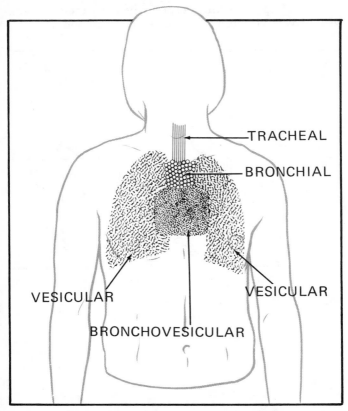

Figure 11-3. Areas of Normal Breath Sounds

Vesicular
  Normal, soft breath sounds.

Bronchial
  Louder, tubular sounds, mostly during expiration.
    Heard at trachea and anterior chest of two main
    bronchi.

Bronchovesicular
  Combination of vesicular and bronchial sounds.
    Heard in upper anterior chest and between
    scapulae on posterior chest.

Note. Deep breathing, especially with mouth open,
will convert vesicular to bronchovesicular sounds.

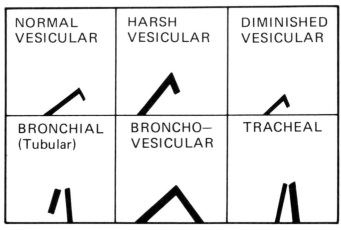

NORMAL VESICULAR	HARSH VESICULAR	DIMINISHED VESICULAR
BRONCHIAL (Tubular)	BRONCHO‑ VESICULAR	TRACHEAL

Figure 11-4. Normal Breath Sounds

Table 11-3   Altered Voice Sounds

Diagnosis	Indications
Bronchophony	Patient says "99" and is normally indistinct on auscultation. May become more distinct with atelectasis or lung consolidation.
Whispered pectoriloquy	Patient whispers "1, 2, 3" which is normally inaudible on auscultation. Increased clarity and volume with lung consolidation.
Egophony	Patient says "e" which normally sounds like "e" on auscultation. With consolidation or pleural effusion the "e" sounds like "a" to the examiner.

Stertorous Respirations
Snoring respirations, usually benign but may be caused by secretions in upper respiratory tract.

Stridulous Respirations
Characterized by high-pitched whistling or crowing sound. Heard in children with croup, foreign body in throat, diptheria membrane or growth in area of vocal chords.

Palpation and Percussion.

Anterior Chest. Palpate anterior of chest for fremitus in a systematic way with open palm of hand on chest wall. Normal vibrations made by breathing should *not* be felt. Ask patient to say "three" and "99" and compare sides for differences in conduction.

Increased conduction in one area may mean consolidation.

Palpate axilla for enlarged lymph nodes.

Note any areas of tenderness or crepitus (subcutaneous emphysema).

Percuss anterior chest in a systematic manner comparing sides as you progress from top to bottom of chest. Note excursion of diaphragm as patient inhales.

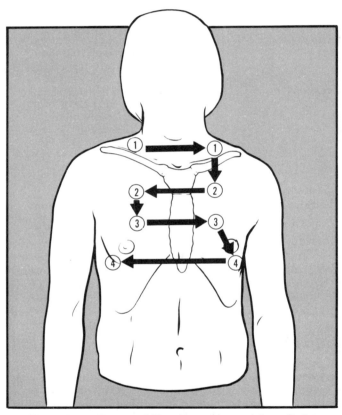

Figure 11-5. Pattern of Chest Percussion and Auscultation

Posterior Chest. Have patient flex head forward and cross arms at waist to separate scapulae.

Percuss posterior chest first with closed fist starting at base of chest and moving toward shoulder to note any rib or muscle tenderness.

Percuss posterior chest in usual manner beginning at the top of the lungs and moving toward the base. Note excursion of diaphragm as patient inhales. Change in resonant area due to diaphragm contraction is usually 3-5 cm. in females and 5-6 cm. in males.

Percussion sounds in chest include:

Resonance: Air-filled lung tissue

Dullness: Less air-filled tissue, more solid tissue such as heart or lung consolidation

Flatness: No air in tissue, solid areas such as spine and liver or pleural effusion

Tympany: Hollow, drum-like sound as over stomach area or large pneumothorax

Auscultation. Auscultate anterior and posterior chest in a systematic manner comparing sides (see diagram above) determining breath sounds, transmission of the whispered voice and abnormal or adventitious sounds. Make careful note of anatomical landmarks (rib number) in relation to lobes of lung in auscultation.

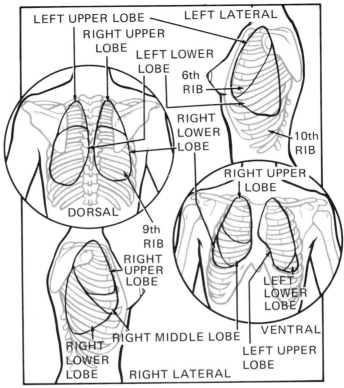

Figure 11-6. Anatomical Relationship of Lung Lobes to Thoracic Cavity

Table 11-4   Adventitious Sounds (Abnormal Sounds)

Diagnosis	Indications
Rales	Sounds in the alveoli and small airways of the lungs caused by movement of secretions, fluid or exudate or passage of air through constricted smaller airways.
Rhonchi	A term which is frequently used interchangeably with rales. Usually refers to coarser sounds due to movement of secretions in narrowed larger airways. Sonorous rhonchi is a snoring sound while sibilant rhonchi means musical or wheezing sound.
Friction Rub	Sound described as rubbing or grating, due to inflammed pleural surfaces as in pleurisy, pneumonia, pulmonary infarction. Occurs with respiration.

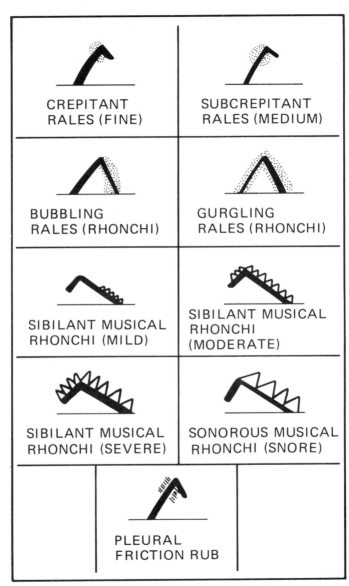

Figure 11-7. Abnormal Breath Sounds

12

CARDIOVASCULAR

Heart

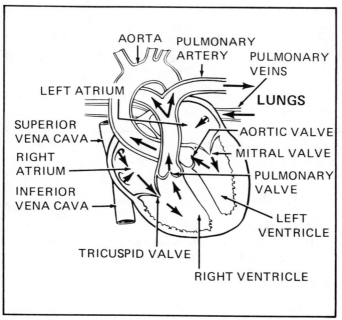

Figure 12-1. Internal Anatomy of the Heart

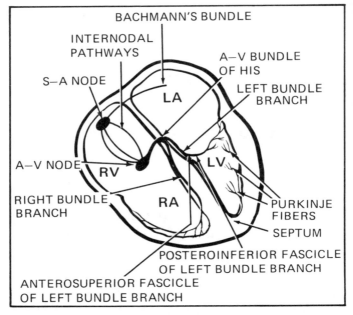

Figure 12-2. Conduction Pathways of the Heart

History Questions

Chest pain
   Description, location, onset, radiation, frequency
   Accompanying symptoms, relief
   Medications

Shortness of breath
   When you first noticed it
   When it bothers you most
   How far can you walk or exercise, number of stairs
   How relieved
   Medication

Difficulty breathing at night
   Number of pillows to sleep, recent change

Cough
When you first noticed it
Productive and description

Changes in heart rate or rhythm

Fatigue
Activities you can no longer perform
Daily rest required

Edema
Recent weight changes
Feet and hands

Extremities
Coldness of extremities, tolerance of temperature changes
Cyanosis, redness or other color changes of extremities
Pain in extremities, description, onset, relieving factors
Ulcers, difficulty healing
Skin texture changes, loss of hair on extremities

Varicose veins
Location, onset
Pain
Use of support hose

Examination

Inspection. Inspect precordium and describe any pulsations, lifts, or rib retractions. Take particular note if apical pulsation is visible. Inspect internal jugular veins of neck, note pulsations and level of distention. No jugular distention should be seen with patient at 45° angle.

Examine nail beds for cyanosis and clubbing.

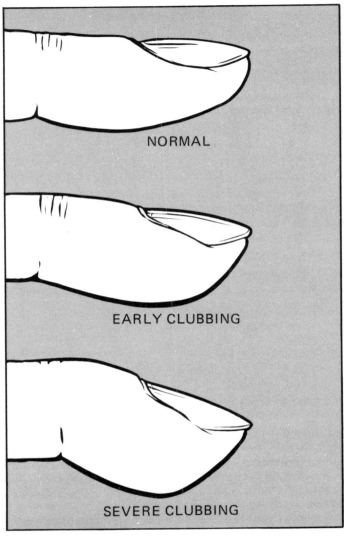

NORMAL

EARLY CLUBBING

SEVERE CLUBBING

Figure 12-3. Fingernail Clubbing

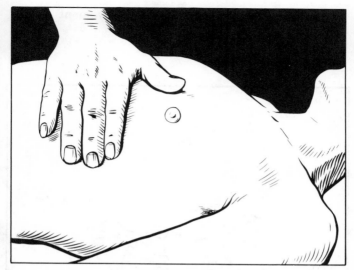

Figure 12-4. Palpation of Precordium

Palpation. Palpate precordium with cushioned part of hand at base of fingers. Proceed in orderly manner from aortic area, pulmonic area, tricuspid area and apical area. Identify point of maximum impulse (PMI) of apical pulse. Record apical pulse by interspace and relationship to midsternal line (MSL) and midclavicular line (MCL). Identify any precordial thrills.

Percussion. Rarely used due to improvement in auscultatory equipment.

Auscultation.

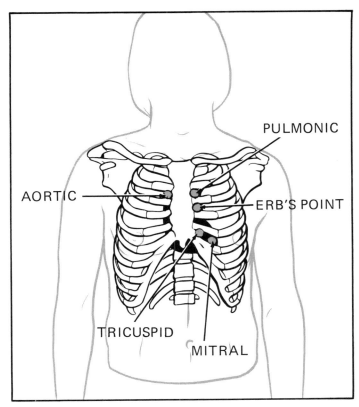

Figure 12-5. Auscultatory Sites

Auscultate at each of the five auscultatory sites in an organized manner. First with the diaphragm of the stethoscope, listen at each site and identify S_1, repeat and identify S_2. Repeat procedure using the bell of the stethoscope, first identify S_1 and S_2, and then extra heart sounds and murmurs, gallops, and friction rubs.

S_1 Contraction of ventricles (systole)
   Closure of mitral and tricuspid valves
   Loudest at apex or mitral area
   Nearly synchronous with carotid pulse
S_2 Relaxation of ventricles (diastole)
   Closure of aortic and pulmonic valve
   Loudest at aortic area
   Physiological splitting may be heard during inspiration
S_3 Heard after S_2 in early diastole
   Bell of stethoscope at apex
   Use left lateral decubitus position
   Normal in healthy children and young adults
   Ventricular gallop
S_4 Heard before S_1, late in diastole
   Bell of stethoscope at apex, also at base
   Atrial gallop
   Represents pathology

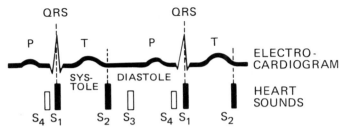

Figure 12-6. Relationship of EKG Complex to Heart Sounds

Special Maneuvers. There are two special maneuvers which should be used to identify or rule out extra heart sounds or murmurs.

Left Lateral Decubitus Position

> Patient is prone and asked to turn 45° to the left side; examiner may support patient's back to maintain this position. Both S_3, S_4 and mitral stenosis may be identified in this position

Far Forward Front Upright

> Patient in a sitting position leans forward, exhales all his air and holds his breath. Stethoscope at 2nd or 3rd intercostal space at left sternal border. Aortic insufficiency is often heard in this position.

Murmurs should be described in the following manner:

Location (anatomical)

Quality
Radiation
Timing (in cardiac cycle)
Loudness

Murmurs should be graded in the following manner:

Grade 1—very soft murmur
Grade 2—easily heard murmur
Grade 3—moderately loud murmur
Grade 4—loud murmur may have accompanying thrill
Grade 5—loud murmur heard with stethoscope barely on chest
Grade 6—loud murmur heard with stethoscope off chest

Below are listed the most common diastolic and systolic murmurs and a description of each.

Systolic Murmurs
Mitral Regurgitation
Location: Apex
Quality: Swoo-sh

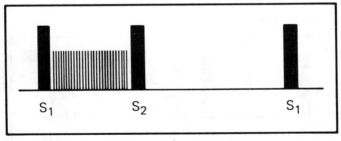

Figure 12-7. Mitral Regurgitation

Radiation: Axilla (except elderly with sclerosis)
Timing: Pansystolic, steady intensity
Aortic Stenosis
Location: Aortic and LSB sometimes apex
Quality: Harsh

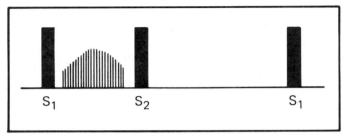

Figure 12-8. Aortic Stenosis

Radiation: Carotid, neck, clavicle
Timing: Systolic, ends before S_2

Diastolic Murmurs
Mitral Stenosis (hardest to hear)
Location: Apex
Quality: Rumble, low pitched
Radiation: None

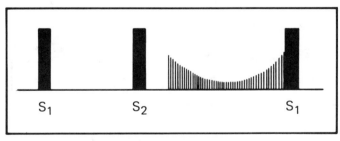

Figure 12-9. Mitral Stenosis

Timing: Early to mid diastole after S_2, before S_3; may need to use special maneuver of left lateral decubitus position

Aortic Insufficiency (Regurgitation)
Location: LLSB, base

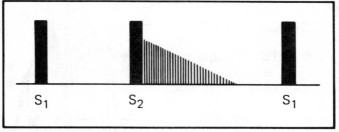

Figure 12-10.   Aortic Regurgitation

Quality: Wind in trees, blowing, high pitched
Radiation: Neck
Timing: In early diastole; may need to use special maneuver with patient upright, forward and all air exhaled

Peripheral Vascular

See following pages.

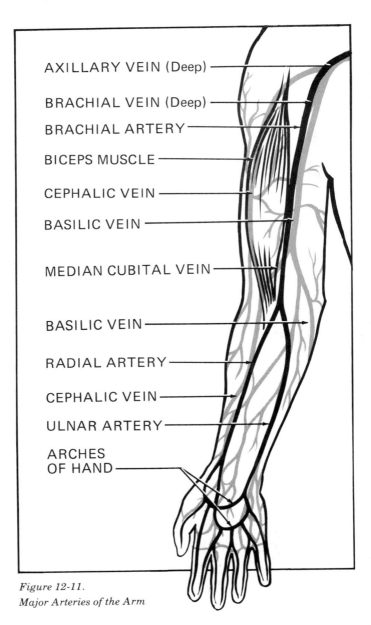

AXILLARY VEIN (Deep)

BRACHIAL VEIN (Deep)

BRACHIAL ARTERY

BICEPS MUSCLE

CEPHALIC VEIN

BASILIC VEIN

MEDIAN CUBITAL VEIN

BASILIC VEIN

RADIAL ARTERY

CEPHALIC VEIN

ULNAR ARTERY

ARCHES
OF HAND

Figure 12-11.
Major Arteries of the Arm

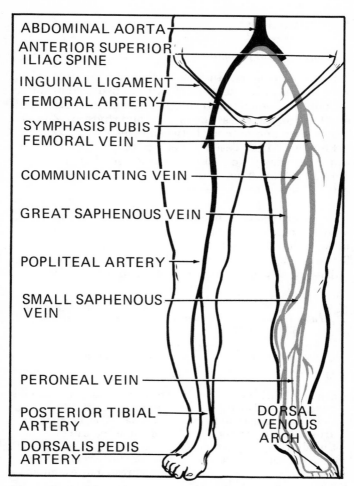

ABDOMINAL AORTA
ANTERIOR SUPERIOR ILIAC SPINE
INGUINAL LIGAMENT
FEMORAL ARTERY
SYMPHASIS PUBIS
FEMORAL VEIN
COMMUNICATING VEIN
GREAT SAPHENOUS VEIN
POPLITEAL ARTERY
SMALL SAPHENOUS VEIN
PERONEAL VEIN
POSTERIOR TIBIAL ARTERY
DORSALIS PEDIS ARTERY
DORSAL VENOUS ARCH

Figure 12-12. Major Veins and Arteries of the Leg

99

Examination

Inspection and Palpation.

Upper Extremities. Inspect both arms, noting color, skin temperature, texture of skin, hair distribution or lack of hair, venous patterns, and edema. Palpate radial and brachial arteries, noting rate and rhythm, comparing volume and patency between sides.

Perform Allen Test to check patency of radial and ulnar arteries if occlusion is suspected. This test is of particular importance in patients requiring frequent arterial punctures for blood gas analysis.

Lower extremities. Inspect legs and feet noting color, skin temperature, texture of skin, hair distribution or lack of hair, venous patterns and edema. Palpate femoral, popliteal, posterior tibial and dorsalis pedis pulses. Note volume, patency and equality of sides.

Table 12-1.   Special Maneuvers to Test Vascular System

Test Maneuver	*Results*
Allen Test. With hand raised, have patient clench fist tightly, occlude radial artery with examiner's thumb. Then have patient open his hand in a relaxed position. Repeat test and occlude ulnar artery to determine patency of radial artery.	The color of the palms should promptly return to a normal color. Persistence of pallor indicates occlusion of the ulnar artery (artery not being compressed by examiner).

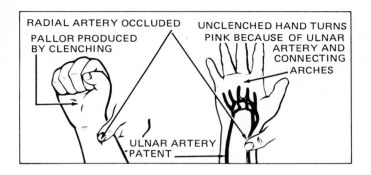

RADIAL ARTERY OCCLUDED
PALLOR PRODUCED
BY CLENCHING

UNCLENCHED HAND TURNS
PINK BECAUSE OF ULNAR
ARTERY AND
CONNECTING
ARCHES

ULNAR ARTERY
PATENT

Elevate both legs 12 inches and move feet up and down at ankles 30–60 seconds.	Maneuver removes venous blood, increased or unusual pallor of extremities indicates poor arterial blood supply to legs, arterial insufficiency.
Following above maneuver have patient sit up and dangle legs.	Color should return in 10 seconds, veins in feet and ankles should fill in 15 seconds. Delay of these indicate poor arterial response.
Homan's Sign. Dorsiflex foot with leg flat on bed.	Presence of calf pain with this maneuver suggests phlebitis.
Squeeze large calf muscles against tibia.	Tenderness, increased firmness, or edema. Suggests deep phlebitis.

13

ABDOMEN

History Questions

Pain in abdomen
  Location, duration, character, quality, association
    factors, aggravating and alleviating factors
  On defecation

Change in appetite
  Weight loss or gain

Chewing and swallowing problems
Heart burn
    Frequency
    Antacids

Nausea, vomiting, regurgitation
Rectal bleeding
    Frequency
    Color: Bright red or tarry stools

Elimination
    Constipation
    Diarrhea
    Change in shape of stool
    Roughage
    Cathartics

Right Upper
  Quadrant
Right lobe of liver
Gallbladder
Pylorus
Duodenum
Head of the pan-
  creas
Upper part of
  right kidney
Hepatic flexure of
  colon

Left Upper Quad-
  rant
Left lobe of liver
Spleen
Stomach
Left kidney
Body and tail of
  pancreas
Splenic flexure of
  colon

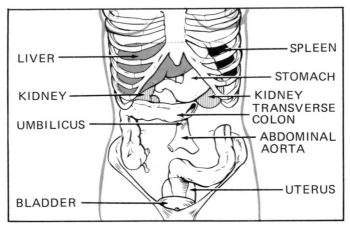

Figure 13-1. Anatomy of Abdominal Cavity

Right Lower
  Quadrant
Lower portion of
  right kidney
Cecum
Appendix
Ascending colon
Right fallopian
  tube
Right ovary
Right ureter

Left Lower Quad-
  rant
Sigmoid colon
Left fallopian
  tube
Left ovary
Left ureter

Midline
Uterus
Urinary bladder

Hemorrhoids
   Pain
   Itching
   Bleeding

Voiding difficulty
   Pain or burning
   Stream
   Nocturia

Previous surgery
   Residual problems

Examination

Inspection. Inspect skin for scars, rashes, lesions, turgor, striae, venous structure, color, petechiae.

Inspect architecture (or contour) and describe:

Protuberant: obese, rounded, distended

Scaphoid: concave, navicular

Symmetry: Masses and deformity will distort; having supine patient lift head off bed will detect ventral hernia.

Inspect umbilicus for protrusion, retraction, discoloration (bluish color may indicate blood in peritoneal cavity), drainage, fistula.

Inspect for pulsations and peristaltic waves.

Auscultation. This technique is performed before percussion and palpation in order to negate alteration of bowel sounds.

Auscultate for evidence of bowel sounds. Use the diaphragm of the stethoscope lightly and listen in all four quadrants. Before reporting the absence of bowel sounds, listen carefully in all quadrants for five minutes.

Evaluate pitch and intensity of sounds. Listen for abnormal sounds which are:

Increased frequency and intensity of bowel sounds (borborygmi) in enteritis or small bowel obstruction

Loud and continuous sounds in bacterial and viral enteritis

Peristaltic rushes and metallic tinkling sounds alternating with periods of silence in bowel obstruction

Rough grating sounds of peritoneal friction rub from an inflammed visceral peritoneum

Auscultate for bruits which are heard most often in cardiac systole. Abdominal bruits are typically soft sounds and can easily be missed. Listen:

Between the xiphoid process and the umbilicus for bruits due to aneurysm of the abdominal aorta.

Over the flank areas or costovertebral angles for renal artery stenosis

Over the liver for the continuous venous hum of cirrhosis

Percussion. Percuss in all four quadrants lightly to assess general proportion and distribution of tympany and dullness.

Percuss the liver:

In the right mid-clavicular line, starting below the umbilicus (and percussing upward toward the liver to determine lower border liver dullness).

In the right mid-clavicular line from lung resonance down toward liver dullness. Measure in centimeters the vertical height of liver dullness

Percussion may outline the liver boundaries in the right mid-sternal area also.

It should be noted that liver heights are generally greater in men than women and in the tall, as opposed to the short, individual.

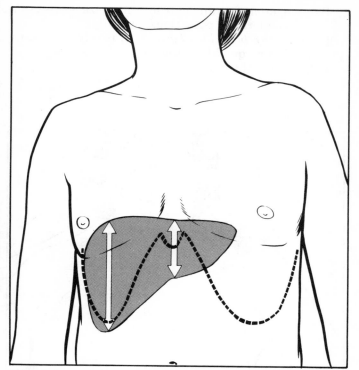

Figure 13-2. Normal Liver Heights

Percuss over the left lower anterior rib cage to identify the tympany of the gastric air bubble.

Percuss for tympany in the lowest interspace in the
left anterior axillary line. Ask the patient to take a deep
breath; if continued percussion reveals the same tympany note, the spleen is probably normal in size.

Palpation. Palpate lightly initially in all four quadrants away from pain to identify abdominal tenderness
and superficial masses. Then palpate deeply in all quadrants to delineate abdominal organs and masses.

Palpate for *masses* and note location, size, shape, consistency, tenderness, pulsations, mobility.

Palpate for *rebound tenderness* (by firmly and slowly pressing in and quickly withdrawing fingers).

Palpation of the liver.

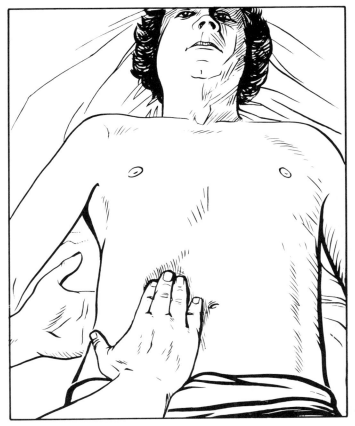

Figure 13-3. Technique for Liver Palpation

Place fingertips below the lower border of liver dullness, pointing toward right costal margin and have the patient take a deep breath. Feel the liver edge as it descends on inspiration.

Scratch test. This test is helpful in determining the location of the liver edge, especially in patients with an enlarged liver. To determine the location of the liver edge, auscultate and simultaneously scratch the abdomen (in small horizontal strokes) beginning at the xiphoid process and progressing to the umbilicus and to the right upper quadrant. A loud, distinct sound will be heard in the area of the liver. The sound disappears as the scratching goes beyond the liver edge.

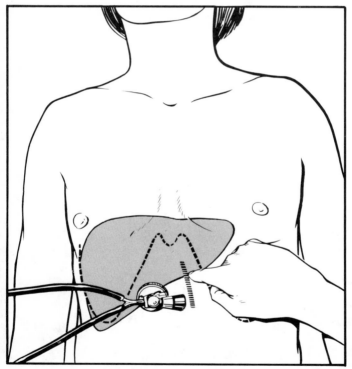

Figure 13-4.   Scratch Test

Palpate in the lower left rib cage for the spleen by placing the patient on the right side with legs bent for gravity to bring spleen into palpable location. The spleen must be enlarged to three times its normal size to be palpable.

Palpate for aortic pulsations in the upper abdomen slightly left to the mid-line.

┤14├

MUSCULOSKELETAL

History Questions

Difficulty with joint movement
Morning stiffness, weakness, related to particular
activity, related to weight bearing

Change in bones or joints
Swelling, inflammation

Change in sensation
Vibratory, temperature, light touch

Leg cramps
At rest, walking, with exercise

Muscle atrophy
Do arms and legs seem to be the same size

General condition
How well do joints and muscles do what they used
to do, ADL

Examination

Inspection and palpation. General approach.

Note active and passive ROM
Note any swelling, deformity
Listen for crepitation or grating as joint moves
Note muscle strength, atrophy, hypertrophy

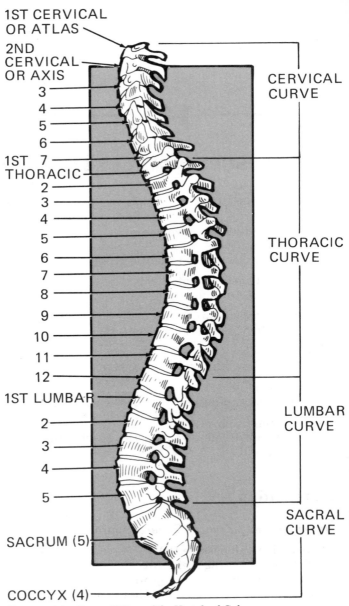

1ST CERVICAL OR ATLAS

2ND CERVICAL OR AXIS

3

4

5

6

1ST 7 THORACIC

2

3

4

5

6

7

8

9

10

11

12

1ST LUMBAR

2

3

4

5

SACRUM (5)

COCCYX (4)

CERVICAL CURVE

THORACIC CURVE

LUMBAR CURVE

SACRAL CURVE

Figure 14-1. Lateral View of the Vertebral Column

112

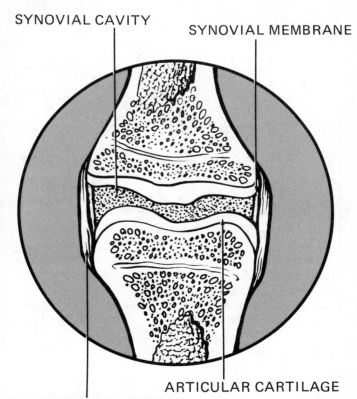

SYNOVIAL CAVITY   SYNOVIAL MEMBRANE

ARTICULAR CARTILAGE

COLLATERAL LIGAMENT

Figure 14-2.   The Basic Structure of a Synovial Joint

Note condition of surrounding tissues, skin changes, subcutaneous nodules
Note symmetry

Back and vertebral column with patient standing

Note *normal curves:* Cervical concavity, thoracic convexity, lumbar concavity
Palpate for tenderness around the spinous processes and paravertebral muscles, note any muscle spasms

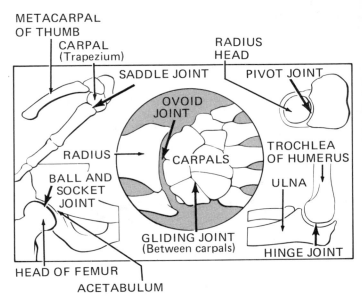

Figure 14-3. *The Six Basic Types of Synovial Joints, Illustrated by Joints of the Body*

Standing behind patient note:
    Any sacral edema
    Lateral curve (scoliosis), if present
    Differences in height of shoulders and iliac crests

With patient touching toes note:
    Symmetry
    Flattening of lumbar curve
    ROM

While stabilizing patient's pelvis, note his ability to bend sideways, bend backwards, twist shoulders.

Head and upper extremities with patient sitting
    Head and neck
    Inspect neck for abonormalities and deformities
    Palpate temporomandibular joint; tenderness around spinous processes and paravertebral muscles

Assess ROM: Flexion, extension, rotation, lateral bending

Hands and Wrists
    Inspect for swelling, redness, nodules, deformities
    Palpate each joint
    Assess ROM: Extend and spread fingers; make fist with thumbs across fingers; flex, extend, abduct and adduct wrists

Elbows
    Inspect around olecranon, and humeral epicondyles
    Palpate around olecranon, and humeral epicondyles
    Assess ROM: Flex, extend, pronate, supinate

Shoulders
    Inspect anteriorly and posteriorly
    Palpate sternoclavicular joint, acromioclavicular joint, entire shoulder
    Assess ROM: Flexion, extension, abuduction, adduction, internal rotation, external rotation

Lower extremities with patient lying down.

Feet and Ankles
    Inspect ankle joint, Achilles' tendon, remaining joints
    Assess ROM: dorsiflexion, plantar flexion, inversion, eversion, flexion and extension of toes

Knees
    Inspect for alignment, status of quadriceps, loss of normal hollows around the patella
    Palpate suprapatellar pouch
    Assess ROM: Flexion and extension

Hips and Pelvis
    Inspect for symmetry
    Assess ROM: With knees flexed—flexion, extension, internal, external rotation; with knees extended-flexion, extension, hyperextension, abduction, adduction. *Note.* These maneuvers should be done with extreme caution on patients who have had recent hip replacements.

Deep Tendon Reflexes

General Principles

Assist patient to relax

Position limb so muscle is mildly stretched

Strike tendon briskly, holding hammer loosely yet controlled

Compare responses in symmetrical manner, side to side

Use following symbols to indicate response:

+ + + +	hyperactive
+ + +	brisker than normal
+ +	normal
+	hypoactive
O	absent

Try *reinforcement techniques* if reflex is difficult to elicit:

Ask patient to contract muscle minimally.

Ask patient to hook fingers together and, on command, pull them in opposite directions while examiner attempts to elicit reflexes of *lower extremities.*

Ask patient to clench one fist tightly while examiner attempts to elicit reflexes in *opposite arm.*

Note. See neurological examination for complete tendon reflex assessment, p. 149

FEMALE GENITALIA AND RECTUM

History Questions

Menses
    Age of menarche
    Cycle description
       Frequency, irregularity
       Amount of flow
    Dysmenorrhea, primary or secondary
    Spotting between periods
    Date of last menstrual period

Menopause
    Age of last menstrual period
    Climacteric symptoms
       Changed, or cessation of, periods, flushing, palpitations,
       Sweats, vaginal dryness
    Changes noted

Sexual
    Pregnancies
       Mode of delivery
       Anesthesia
       Problems, complications
       Birth weight of children
       Problem getting pregnant
       Type of contraception

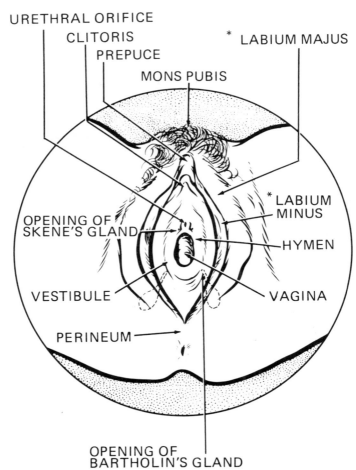

URETHRAL ORIFICE
CLITORIS
PREPUCE
MONS PUBIS
* LABIUM MAJUS
* LABIUM MINUS
HYMEN
OPENING OF SKENE'S GLAND
VESTIBULE
VAGINA
PERINEUM
OPENING OF BARTHOLIN'S GLAND

* (Labia are separated for visualization of structures between them)

Figure 15-1. Exterior Anatomy of Female Genitalia

118

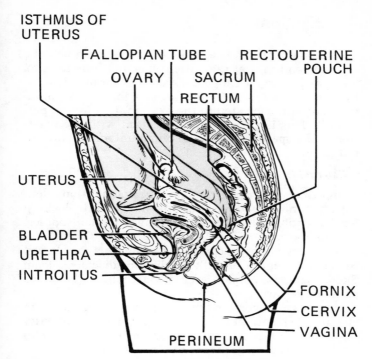

Figure 15-2.   Interior Anatomy of Female Genitalia

Labels on figure:
ISTHMUS OF UTERUS
FALLOPIAN TUBE
OVARY
SACRUM
RECTUM
RECTOUTERINE POUCH
UTERUS
BLADDER
URETHRA
INTROITUS
PERINEUM
FORNIX
CERVIX
VAGINA

    Bleeding or pain during intercourse (dyspareunia)
    Satisfactory sexual adjustment

General
   Douching practices
   Last Pap test and result
   Discharge
   Medications

Examination

This part of the physical examination should be done near the end so that the patient has had time to relax and establish some rapport with the examiner. The patient should have an empty bladder for the examination. Explain each step in the examination as you perform it. This is particularly important with the insertion of the speculum, and the bimanual and rectovaginal exams.

External Genitalia

Inspection and Palpation. Note hair distribution, identify anatomical landmarks of external genitalia looking for lacerations, lesions, edema, hematomas, masses, and discharge.

With gloved hand separate the labia majora. Insert finger into vagina to milk urethra for discharge from Skene's glands, palpate area of Bartholin's glands for pain or discharge.

Move two fingers inside the vagina and separate opening. Ask patient to bear down and observe for bulging of the anterior (cystocele) or posterior (rectocele) wall of the vagina or incontinence of urine.

Internal Genitalia

Inspection (speculum exam). A speculum of the proper size should be lubricated and warmed by running warm water over it (commonly used jelly lubricants can interfere with results of Pap test or other cytological studies.)

Insertion of speculum utilizing following steps:

1. Place two fingers (R hand) just inside or at introitus of vagina, gently pressing down.

2. Introduce closed speculum (L hand) past fingers at 45° angle down and posteriorly holding blades vertically.

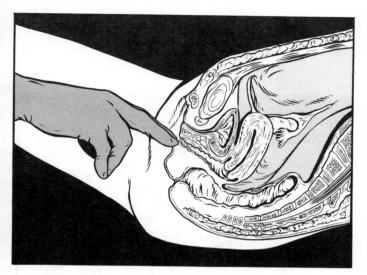

Figure 15-3. Fingers at Introitus of Vagina

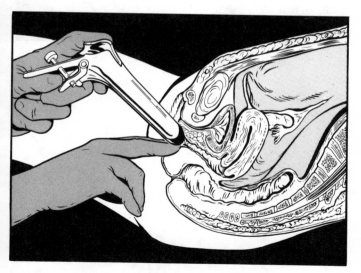

Figure 15-4. Insertion of Speculum

3. Advance speculum by putting pressure on posterior vaginal wall.
4. After speculum has entered vagina, remove fingers and rotate blades to horizontal position.

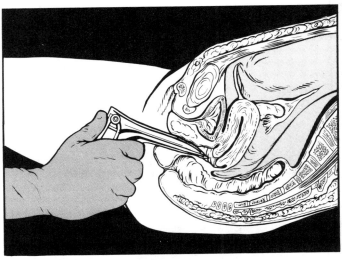

Figure 15-5. Rotation of Speculum Blades to Horizontal Position

5. Open the blades after full insertion and maneuver until cervix is in full view.

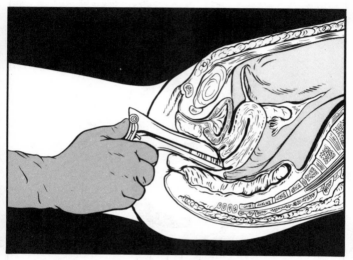

Figure 15-6.   Opening of Speculum Blades

6. Adjust speculum to remain in open position.

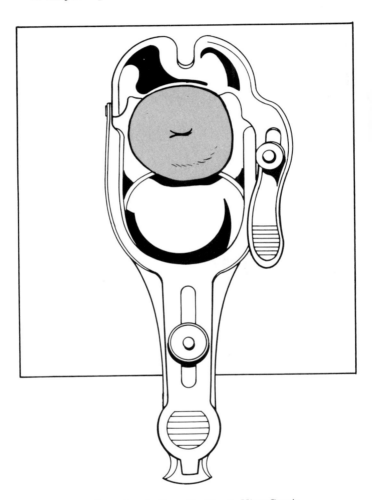

Figure 15-7. Speculum in Open Position to View Cervix

Inspect *vagina* for color, discharge, lesions.

Inspect *cervix* for description of os, color, erosions, lacerations, and discharge.

Perform *Papanicolaou Test* for cervical cytology if part of examination.

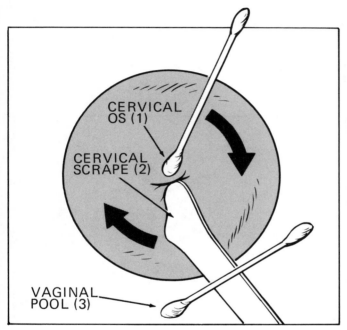

Figure 15-8.   Papanicolaou Test

1. Cervical os. Insert cotton-tipped applicator into opening of cervix. Roll between fingers to pick up discharge. Smear gently onto glass slide. Use proper fixation agent immediately.
2. Cervical scrape. With special spatula, place long end into cervical os and rotate spatula around entire cervical opening in a scraping manner. Smear

spatula onto glass slide. Use proper fixation agent immediately.

3. Vaginal Pool. Insert cotton-tipped applicator into posterior fornix, vaginal pool below cervix. Smear gently onto glass slide. Use proper fixation agent immediately.

Note. The inside of the cervix is lined with columnar epithelium; the outside of the cervix is covered with squamous epithelium. Most cancers begin at the squamo-columnar junction near the cervical os. Proper scraping of cells at this area is vital to proper cytology tests.

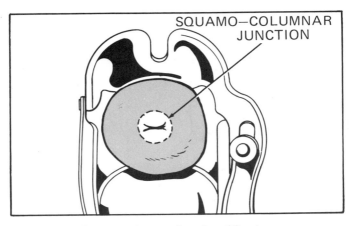

Figure 15-9. Squamo-columnar Junction of Cervix

If cervix has been surgically removed, perform a scrape from the vaginal cuff and a specimen from the vaginal pool.

Table 15-1. *Common Vaginal Discharges*

Characteristics of Discharge	Patient Symptoms	Probable Causes
Clear discharge changing to thick white viscous discharge	None	Normal First two weeks after menses discharge is clear changing to thicker white after ovulation.
Thick white curd-like or cheesy appearance, discharge, adheres to vaginal wall, usually little odor	Itching, inflamed vulva	Monilia (candida) treated with vaginal suppositories. This is a yeast infection and symptomatic relief enhanced with baking soda douches.
Profuse yellow or greenish-gray, often frothy and foul smelling discharge, vaginal wall and cervix (strawberry spots) may have red granular or petechiae spots.	Profuse, foul discharge, itching, inflamed vulva.	Trichomonas vaginalis. Treated with oral medication and should consider treating patient's sexual partner to prevent "ping-pong" effect of reinfection.
Yellow to greenish discharge often with inflamed urethra and Bartholin's glands. Cervix may be inflamed and yellowish discharge from os.	Change in vaginal discharge and painful urination.	Gonorrhea treated routinely with penicillin unless patient is allergic. Sexual partner(s) must be treated also.

127

Thin, whitish, bloodtinged discharge. No external inflammation.	Vaginal dryness, painful intercourse, often with bleeding	Atrophic (senile) vaginitis. Treat with vaginal cream or low level hormones.

Palpation. Bimanual Exam. The examiner is in a standing position, inserts gloved and lubricated index and middle fingers with pressure on posterior surface. Turn finger pads to face anterior wall. Palpate vaginal wall. Note firmness, tenderness, masses, bulging of wall.

Palpate *cervix.* Note contour, tenderness, mobility, masses or nodules.

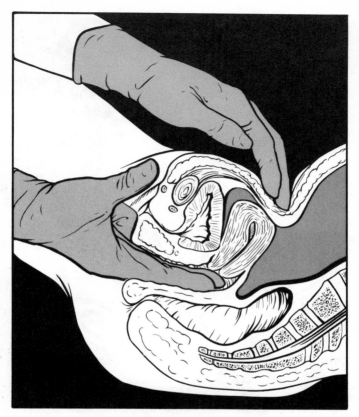

Figure 15-10. Palpation of Cervix

Palpate *uterus* by pressing downward on abdominal wall with outside hand while pushing upward on either side of cervix with two fingers in vagina. Bimanually palpate uterus. Note size, shape, position, consistency, mobility, and tenderness.

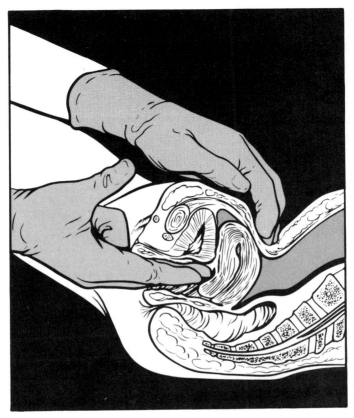

Figure 15-11. Bimanual Palpation of Uterus

Palpate *ovaries* by pressing downward with hand on abdomen and upward with fingers in vagina at each side of uterus. This should be a stroking motion with the fingers of both hands pushing together as the hands are moved downward. Note size, shape, mobility, and tenderness.

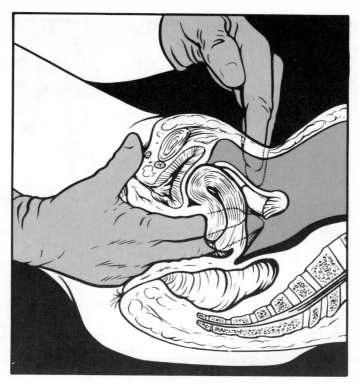

Figure 15-12.   Bimanual Palpation of Ovaries

Rectovaginal exam. Change gloves and lubricate index and middle finger. Insert index finger into vagina, the middle finger into rectum. Repeat maneuvers of bimanual exam with special attention to area in rectum behind cervix. Remove fingers. Use stool on glove of middle finger to perform test for occult blood (guaiac).

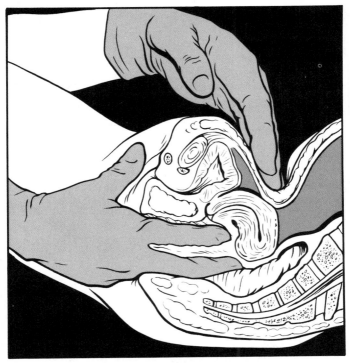

Figure 15-13. Rectovaginal Examination

|16|

MALE GENITALIA AND RECTUM

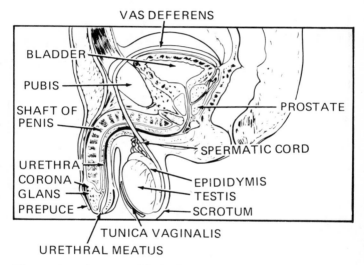

Figure 16-1. Anatomy of the Male Genitalia

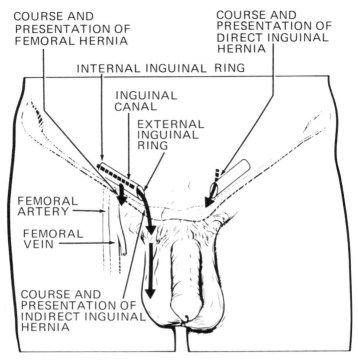

COURSE AND PRESENTATION OF FEMORAL HERNIA

COURSE AND PRESENTATION OF DIRECT INGUINAL HERNIA

INTERNAL INGUINAL RING

INGUINAL CANAL

EXTERNAL INGUINAL RING

FEMORAL ARTERY

FEMORAL VEIN

COURSE AND PRESENTATION OF INDIRECT INGUINAL HERNIA

Figure 16-2. Hernias in the Groin

History Questions

Problems with urination
  Frequency, urgency, stream, nocturia, incontinence, pain

Testicular changes
  Tenderness, pain, change in size

Evidence of hernia
  Visible bulging

Rectal problems
   Stool color
   Bleeding, constipation, hemorrhoids

Sexual difficulty
   Changes, impotence

Examination

The techniques of inspection and palpation are utilized to examine the male genitalia. Use of gloves by the examiner is a reasonable practice.

Inspection and Palpation. Inspect and palpate the following structures:

Penis. Note hair distribution, size, shape, color, lesions, edema, nodules. Ask the patient to retract the prepuce and note glands for hygiene, size and placement of urethral meatus, discharge, lesions.

Scrotum. Note general size, contour, skin color (normally the left side is larger than the right). Spread walls of scrotum between fingers and note lesions, nodules. Lift scrotum to inspect posterior surface. Using thumbs and forefingers compare content of each scrotal side.

Identify the testes noting consistency, size shape, tenderness, nodules, symmetry; the epididymis on the posterior surface of the testes noting symmetry, tenderness, size, shape. Grasp spermatic cord on each side, at neck of scrotum, between thumb and forefinger. Palpate length of cord down to testes. Note any masses or thickening.

Transilluminate any swelling. Hold pen light behind the scrotal content. Serous fluid will transilluminate; blood and tissue will not.

Hernias. With the patient standing, inspect inguinal and femoral regions for scars, lesions, enlarged lymph nodes, hernia bulges. Ask patient to strain to accentuate bulges.

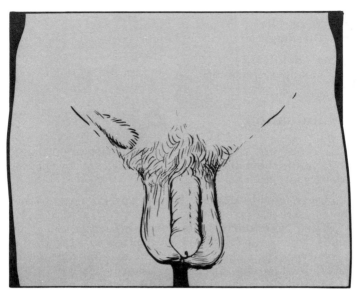

Figure 16-3. Indirect hernia commonly seen in middle of inguinal area

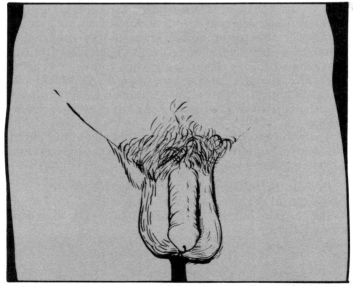

Figure 16-4. Direct hernia commonly seen near the symphysis

136

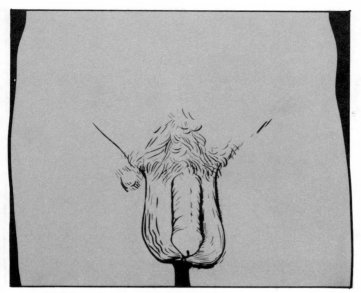

Figure 16-5. Femoral hernia commonly seen below the inguinal ligament, near the symphysis

Palpate the inguinal canal by invaginating loose fold of the scrotal sac into the external inguinal ring with the fingertip. Ask the patient to strain. An indirect hernia will come down the inguinal canal and touch or tap the fingertip. A direct hernia will bulge anteriorly and push the side of the finger forward.

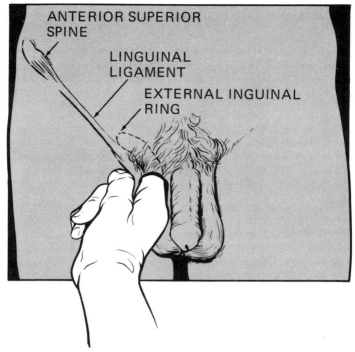

Figure 16-6. Palpation of the Inguinal Canal

Rectum. With patient standing and leaning over the examining table (for non-ambulatory patients the left lateral position with the right knee flexed is preferred.), inspect the sacrococcygeal and perineal areas for inflammation, lesions, lumps. Spread the buttocks to inspect the anal area for external hemorrhoids, skin tags, rashes, scars, fissures, fistulas. Ask the patient to bear down. Note any hemorrhoids or tags. Place pad of lubricated finger over the anus and as sphincter relaxes, insert fingertip into anal canal.

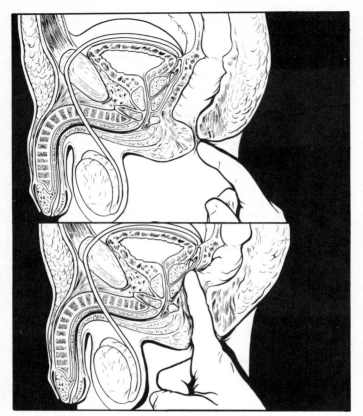

Figure 16-7. Insertion of Fingertip into Rectum

Direct finger toward umbilicus and note sphincter tone, tenderness, irregularities. Palpate the right lateral, posterior, and left lateral surfaces, noting any irregularities. Palpate the anterior surface identifying the lateral lobes and median sulcus of the prostate gland. Note size, shape, consistency, nodularity, tenderness. Withdraw finger from rectum and test any fecal material for occult blood (guaiac).

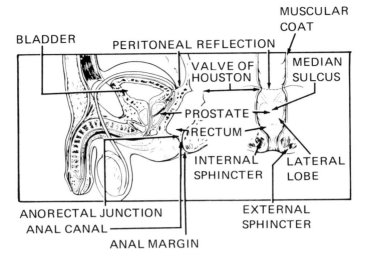

Figure 16-8. Male Anus and Rectum

NEUROLOGICAL

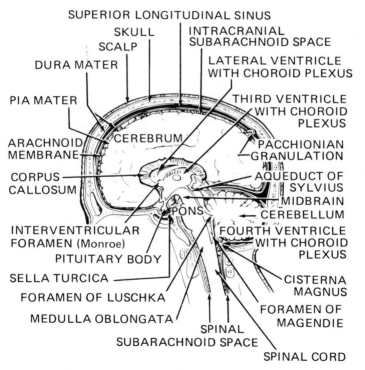

SUPERIOR LONGITUDINAL SINUS
SKULL
SCALP
DURA MATER
PIA MATER
ARACHNOID MEMBRANE
CORPUS CALLOSUM
INTERVENTRICULAR FORAMEN (Monroe)
PITUITARY BODY
SELLA TURCICA
FORAMEN OF LUSCHKA
MEDULLA OBLONGATA

INTRACRANIAL SUBARACHNOID SPACE
LATERAL VENTRICLE WITH CHOROID PLEXUS
THIRD VENTRICLE WITH CHOROID PLEXUS
PACCHIONIAN GRANULATION
AQUEDUCT OF SYLVIUS
MIDBRAIN
CEREBELLUM
FOURTH VENTRICLE WITH CHOROID PLEXUS
CISTERNA MAGNUS
FORAMEN OF MAGENDIE

CEREBRUM
PONS
SPINAL SUBARACHNOID SPACE
SPINAL CORD

Figure 17-1. Main Anatomical Structure of the Brain

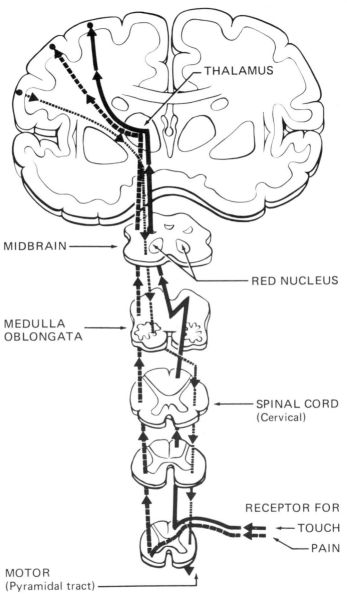

THALAMUS

MIDBRAIN

RED NUCLEUS

MEDULLA
OBLONGATA

SPINAL CORD
(Cervical)

RECEPTOR FOR
— TOUCH
— PAIN

MOTOR
(Pyramidal tract)

Figure 17-2. Main Motor and Sensory Pathways

History Questions

Headaches
    Description, character, frequency
    Onset, accompanying symptoms
    Relief, medications

Vertigo, syncope, convulsions

Paralysis, paresthesias, neuralgia
    Description, location, onset

Memory and orientation
    Short and long term
    Amnesia episodes

Visual difficulties
    Double vision, areas of blindness
    Loss of eye movement

Facial Weakness
    Drooping eyelid, cheek, mouth

Difficulty swallowing, with speech

Difficulty with handling saliva, drooling

Difficulty with head and neck movements

Examination

The neurological examination is accomplished primarily through observing the patient in performing normal activities and some special maneuvers to detect deficits. The neurological examination is done near the end of the physical because many of the elements of the examination have already been performed, but an organized summary should be completed with any additional findings. The components of the neurological examination include the following.

Cerebral Function
    Mental status, level of consciousness, short and long term memory.

Emotional status, affect and mood.
Cognitive abilities, coherency and thought process, abstract reasoning.
Behavior, appropriateness of responses, dress and grooming, facial expressions, speech.

Cranial Nerves

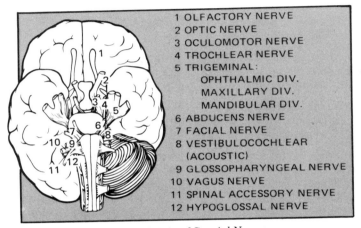

1 OLFACTORY NERVE
2 OPTIC NERVE
3 OCULOMOTOR NERVE
4 TROCHLEAR NERVE
5 TRIGEMINAL:
   OPHTHALMIC DIV.
   MAXILLARY DIV.
   MANDIBULAR DIV.
6 ABDUCENS NERVE
7 FACIAL NERVE
8 VESTIBULOCOCHLEAR
   (ACOUSTIC)
9 GLOSSOPHARYNGEAL NERVE
10 VAGUS NERVE
11 SPINAL ACCESSORY NERVE
12 HYPOGLOSSAL NERVE

Figure 17-3.   Anatomy of Origin of Cranial Nerves

Assessment of the cranial nerves is properly a part of the neurological examination. However, the 12 pairs of cranial nerves innervate the structures of the head and neck and are, therefore, tested in the physical examination of the head and neck. If the cranial nerve examination was not recorded after the head and neck exam, it should be completed and recorded at this time.

The cranial nerves are listed below with the proper function and test for each nerve. Each nerve is also labeled indicating whether it has sensory or motor function or both.

Table 17-1. *Assessment of Cranial Nerve Function*

Cranial Nerve	Function	Test
I. Olfactory (S)	Smell	Identifies familiar odors as coffee, cloves, mint.
II. Optic (S)	Visual Fields Visual Acuity	Gross confrontation test with penlight or wiggling fingers. Snellen eye chart
III. Oculomotor (M)	Pupil constriction Accommodation Movement of eye muscle (Superior Rectus, Inferior Oblique; Inferior Rectus, Medial Rectus)	With penlight check for constriction and consensual constriction. Check pupil change of near and far objects. Extraocular Movement (EOM)

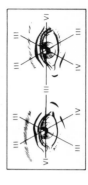

Cranial Nerve	Function	Assessment
		Check EOM of each eye for 3, 4, and 6 cranial nerves
IV. Trochlear (M)	Movement of eye muscle (Superior Oblique)	EOM (see drawing above)
V. Trigeminal (M)	Jaw muscles and muscles of mastication	Open and close jaw tightly.
(S)	Ophthalmic: forehead cornea Maxillary: cheek Mandibular: jaw, mucous membrane of mouth	Identify sharp and dull sensations by pin prick on each area with eyes closed. If pain sensation lost, test temperature sensation. Test corneal reflex with cotton wisp.
VI. Abducens (M)	Movement of eye muscle (Lateral Rectus).	EOM (see drawing above)
VII. Facial (M)	Movement of muscles of face and scalp	Frown, smile, puff cheeks, close eyes tightly.
(S)	Taste anterior ⅔ tongue	Often deferred unless neurological problem. Then have patient identify familiar taste—mint, coffee, salt.
VIII. Acoustic (S)	Cochlear: hearing	Weber Test Rinné Test
	Vestibular: equilibrium	Romberg Test

Nerve	Function	Testing
IX. Glossopharyngeal (S)	Taste posterior ⅓ tongue Pain, touch and temperature in pharynx & throat	Usually deferred unless neurological problem.
(M)	Muscles of pharynx	
X. Vagus (M)	Sensation in larynx, trachea, lungs, esophagus Slows heart, contracts bronchial muscles.	Test together by testing gag reflex, swallowing, and phonation.
XI. Spinal Accessory (M)	Muscles of head and upper shoulders	Rotation of head against resistance. Raise or shrug shoulders against resistance.
XII. Hypoglossal (M)	Tongue movement	Protrude tongue, note tremors or deviation. Push tongue against cheeks.

Cerebellar Function
Coordination-Balance
> Fingers to nose
>> His nose, your finger
>
> Heel to shin or big toe to finger
>> His toe, your finger
>
> Rapid alternating movements
> Gait
>> Walk straight line heel to toe—tandem walking
>
> Romberg
>> Have patient stand with feet together and arms out with *eyes open*. If patient loses balance, this indicates inner ear (vestibular) problem or cerebellar ataxia. If balanced with eyes open, have patient *close eyes* to test sensory equilibrium. Dysfunction will be imbalance (+ Romberg).

Findings that may indicate cerebellar dysfunction:

Tremors
> Resting tremors: Often present in Parkinsonism and go away with action
>
> Intention tremors: No tremors at rest, tremors occur and increase with intentional action

Ataxia
Inability to perform rapid alternating movement
Nystagmus
Speech difficulty
Difficulty swallowing

Most common reasons for cerebellar dysfunction.

Senility
Remote effects of carcinoma
Alcoholism

Motor System
This portion of the neurological exam may have already been done as part of the musculoskeletal exam. If so, do not repeat exam, just refer to musculoskeletal exam.

148

Symmetry of muscle size (side to side comparison) look for loss of muscle mass, especially between fingers and at temporalis muscle.

Muscle tone
Look for spasticity, uncoordination, flaccidity, rigidity

Muscle strength
Test upper extremities by extensor muscles
Wrist and arm: Extend against resistance
Test lower extremities by flexor muscles
Knee bend against resistance
Pull heel toward buttocks against resistance
Pull toes of foot toward nose against resistance

Voluntary muscle dysfunction usually involves the pyramidal spinal tract

Involuntary muscle movement usually involves the extrapyramidal spinal tracts and includes:
Ticks
Myoclonus
Dystonia
Chorea
Fasciculation
Tremors

Problems with muscle strength and function can be caused by:
Muscle disease
Dysfunction or problems of the neuromuscular junction
Peripheral disease: Cut motor fibers to muscles
Spinal cord lesion or disruption
Cerebral lesion of pyramidal tract

In trying to determine upper motor neuron symptoms from lower motor neuron symptoms, the following is helpful:

Table 17-2. Upper and Lower Motor Neuron Symptoms

Upper Motor Neuron Lesion	Lower Motor Neuron Lesion
1. Spastic paralysis (knocks out inhibiting fibers to muscles)	1. Flaccid paralysis
2. Exaggerated deep tendon reflexes	2. Absence of deep tendon reflexes
3. No muscle atrophy	3. Atrophy of muscles
4. Positive Babinski	4. Normal Babinski
5. No fasciculations, cog wheel rigidity	5. Fasciculation due to degeneration of myoneural junction
6. Motor involvement to *opposite* side from brain lesion	6. Motor involvement *same* side as lesion

Sensory System
With *eyes closed* the patient should be able to:
Interpret sensations correctly
Discriminate side to side
Discriminate proximal to distal

Determine if a primary or secondary sensory deficit exists, describe it and sketch where it is.
Primary Sensory Functions (Patient's *eyes closed)*
Tactile: Cotton wisp, may go so far as to check perianal and perineal areas
Superficial pain: Use safety pin, distinguish sharp from dull
Deep pain: Calf, biceps, trapezius (if necessary)
Vibratory: Tuning fork on bony prominences (many neuro deficits are distal first)
Position sense: Move patient's finger up or down to see if he can discern this. Repeat with toes.

150

Temperature: Rarely used

Secondary or Cortical Functions (These tests combine coordination ability with cerebral ability to interpret. Have patient *close his eyes.*)

Stereognosis: Put object such as coin in hand and have patient identify it.

Graphesthesia: Write number or letter of alphabet in palm of patient's hand and have him identify it.

Point location: Touch on forearm, identify location.

Two-point discrimination: Determine "extinction"—touch on both sides of body to see if input from one side makes other side extinct, also how close two points are together before felt as one point.

Reflexes

The reflex response is the contraction of a specific muscle when the tendon of insertion is suddenly stretched by a light tap with the finger or reflex hammer. The grading of the muscle response is usually recorded in the following manner:

Grade 0	0	Absent
Grade 1	+	Diminished but present
Grade 2	++	Normal
Grade 3	+++	Brisker than normal
Grade 4	++++	Hyperactive (Clonus)

The reflexes usually checked included the tendon reflexes and the superficial reflexes.

Table 17-3. Deep Tendon Reflexes

Tendon Reflexes	Nerve Root Tested	
Achilles	S_1, S_2	
Patella	L_2, L_3, L_4	
Biceps and Brachoradialis	C_5, C_6	
Triceps	C_6, C_7, C_8	

151

Table 17-4. Superficial Reflexes

Tendon Reflexes	Nerve Root Tested
Upper Abdominal reflex (stroke ↑ upper abdomen, umbilicus pulls to stimulated side.)	T_7, T_8, T_9
Lower Abdominal Reflex (stroke ↓ lower abdomen, umbilicus pulls to stimulated side.)	T_{10}, T_{11}
Cremasteric reflex (stroke inner thigh, scrotum goes ↑)	T_{12}, L_1, L_2
Plantar (Babinski) (with sharp object stroke lateral sole of foot from heel to ball of foot and across ball of foot.)	S_1, S_2 A positive response is dorsiflexion of the big toe with fanning of the other toes and shows pyramidal tract disease.

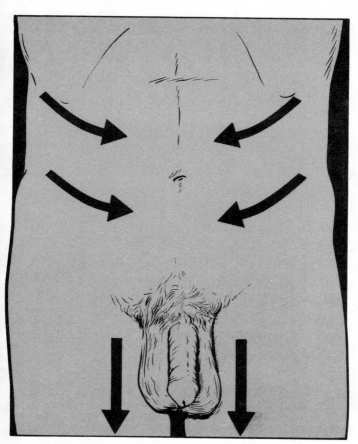

Figure 17-4. Superficial Reflexes

|18|

SELECTED LABORATORY FINDINGS

Table 18-1. Complete Blood Count

Test	Normal Values	Selected Abnormalities
Red Blood Cells (RBC)	Male 4.5-6.0 million/cmm Female 4.0-5.5 million/cmm	↑Polycythemia vera ↑Severe dehydration ↓Hemodilution after blood loss ↓Anemia (see RBC indices)
Hemoglobin (Hgb)	Male 14-18gm/100 ml Female 12-16gm/100 ml	↑Severe dehydration, hemoconcentration ↓Anemia, leukemia
Hematocrit (Hct)	Male 40-54% Female 37-47% Generally Hct = 3X Hgb ± 3%	Same as above
Reticulocyte Count	0.5-1.5% 25,000-75,000 cell/ml	↑Bone marrow hyperproliferative, i.e., hemolytic

		anemia, lymphocytic leukemia, systemic lupus
		↓Bone marrow hypoproliferative, i.e., iron deficiency, pernicious anemia, folic acid deficiency
Erythrocyte Indices Indirect Mean Corpuscular Volume (MCV)	82-92m	↑Macrocytic anemia, i.e., folic acid deficiency, pernicious anemia ↑Normocytic anemia, i.e., chronic renal failure, cancer, acute or chronic infections, chronic liver disease ↓Microcytic anemia, i.e., iron deficiency anemia
Mean Corpuscular Hemoglobin Weight of $\frac{Hgb}{RBC}$ RBC	27-31%	↑Macrocytic anemia (rarely used) ↓Microcytic anemia
Mean Corpuscular Hemoglobin MCHC $\frac{Hgb}{Hct}$ %	32-36%	Normal value = normochromic Low Value = hypochromic
White Blood Count (WBC)	5,000-10,000/ml	↑Acute infections ↓Agranulocytosis (see differential for more specific information)

Table 18-2. W & B Differential

Differential	Relative Value	Absolute Value (WBC X Rel. Val.)	Selected Abnormalities
Neutrophils (in order of development stages)			↑Infection, granulocytic leukemia
Myeloblasts	0	0	↓Mumps, measles, hepatitis, anticonvulsants, antihistamines, sulfonamides, some antibiotics, aplastic anemia, agranulocytosis
Premyelocytes	0	0	
Myelocytes	0	0	
Metamyelocytes	0	0	
Band (non-segmented neutrophils)	0-10%	0-1,000	
Segmented neutrophils	60-70%	3,000-7,000/cmm	
Monocytes	2-6%	100-600/cmm	↑T.B., bacterial endocarditis, monocytic leukemia
Lymphocytes	20-40%	1,000-4,000/cmm	↑(Many viral infections) mumps, german measles, infectious mononeucleosis, viral hepatitis, lymphocytic leukemia ↓Stress from trauma, burns, epinephrine, ACTH, cortisone

157

Differential	Relative Value	Absolute Value (WBC X Rel. Val.)	Selected Abnormalities
Eosinophils	1-4%	50-400/cmm	↑Allergies, asthma, skin diseases ↓High levels of insulin, epinephrine, ACTH
Basophils	0.5-1%	25-100/cmm	↑Granulocytic leukemia, irradiation, hemolytic anemias, splenectomy

Table 18-3. Electrolytes

Tests	Normal Values	Selected Abnormalities
Sodium	136-142 meq/l	↑Decrease water intake ↑Excessive oral or I.V. intake of sodium ↑Diabetes insipidus ↑Sodium bicarbonate given in cardiac arrest ↓GI suctioning ↓Vomiting ↓Diarrhea ↓Adrenal insufficiency ↓Excessive infusion of nonelectrolytes
Potassium	3.5-5 meq/L	↑Renal failure ↑Following severe burn ↑Blood sample left sitting too long ↑Adrenal insufficiency ↓Metabolic and respiratory alkalosis ↓G.I. Loss—diarrhea, vomiting, NG suctioning ↓Potassium wasting drug therapy
CO_2 combining power	24-30 meq/l	See bicarbonate under blood gases.

Chloride	95-103 meq/l	↑Acute renal failure
		↑Renal tubular acidosis
		↓Congestive heart failure
		↓Diarrhea
		↓Adrenal cortical insufficiency

Table 18-4.   Blood Chemistry

Tests	Normal Values	Selected Abnormalities
Amylase	60-160 (Somogyi units)/100 ml	↑Pancreatic disease
Alkaline phosphatase	30-85 IU	↑Post hepatic obstruction ↑Viral hepatitis ↑Infectious mononeucleosis ↑Metastatic bone cancer
Acid phosphatase	0-1.5 U	↑Acute and chronic renal disease ↑Accompanies high alkaline phosphatase in metastatic prostatic carcinoma
BUN (Blood urea nitrogen)	8-18 mg/dl	↑Renal failure ↑Dehydration ↑GI hemorrhage ↑Congestive heart failure ↓Cirrhosis of liver

Calcium	9.0-11.0mg/dl (4.5-5.5meg/L)	↑Primary hyper- parathyroidism ↑Cancer of lung, kidneys ↑Hyperproteinemia ↑Acidosis ↓Low albumin levels ↓Hypoparathyroidism ↓Alkalosis
Creatinine	.6-1.2mg/dl	↑Congestive heart failure ↑Chronic glomerulo-nephritis
Cholesterol	150-250mg/dl	↑Cardiovascular disease ↑Hypothyroidism ↑Nephrosis ↑Uncontrolled dia- betes ↑Obstructive jaun- dice ↓Portal cirrhosis
Triglycerides	10-190mg/dl	↑Uncontrolled dia- betes ↑Obstructive jaun- dice ↓Portal cirrhosis
Total Bilirubin	.2-1.2mg/dl	↑Hemolytic jaun- dice ↑Hepatic jaundice ↑Post hepatic obstructive jaun- dice
Conjugated (di- rect) bilirubin	.1-.2mg/100ml	↑Marked in post hepatic obstructive jaundice ↑Normal in hemolytic jaundice

Unconjugated (indirect) bilirubin	.1-.6mg/100ml	↑In hemolytic jaundice
Uric Acid	Male 2.1-7.8mg/dl Female 2.0-6.4mg/dl	↑Gout ↑Infectious mononucleosis ↑Chemotherapy for cancer ↑Renal failure
Proteins (Total)	6.0-7.8gm/dl	↑Lupus erythematosus ↑Acute liver disease
Albumin	3.2-4.5gm/dl	↓Inadequate protein intake ↓Nephrosis ↓Burns ↓Portal cirrhosis
Globulin	2.3-3.5gm/dl	↑Portal cirrhosis ↑Multiple myeloma

Table 18-5.   Enzymes

Tests	Normal Values	Selected Abnormalities
CPK (creatine phosphokinase)	Male 20-90 IU/L Female 14-60 IU/L	↑Within 4 hours post myocardial infarction ↑Muscular dystrophy ↑Muscle trauma
LDH (lactic dehydrogenase)	80-120 (Weeker units) 150-450 (Wroblewski units)	↑Within a day and peaks in 4 days post myocardial infarction

SGOT (serum glutamic oxyloacetic transaminase)	8.33U/ml	↑Acute liver disease ↑Acute renal disease ↑Acute myocardial infarction
Glucose	70-110mg/dl	↑Diabetes mellitus ↑Brain trauma ↓Excess insulin administered to diabetic ↓Psychogenic conditions
Phosphorus	3-4.5mg/100ml	↑Chronic nephritis ↓Renal tubular acidosis

Table 18-6.   Urinalysis

Test	Normal Values	Selected Abnormalities
Bacteria count Color pH	yellow, clear 4.6-8.0	If shows ↑ bacteria with no WBC's, redo test.
Specific gravity	1.016-1.022 (normal fluid) 1.001-1.035 (range)	If shows ↑ bacterial with WBC's, do a culture and sensitivity.
Glucose	0 neg.	
Albumin	0 neg.	
Blood, occult	0 neg.	
WBC's	0	
Bacteria	0	Usually treat if bacteria > 100,000 and WBC's present.
Total volume/ 24 hr.	600-1600 cc.	

Urine urobilinogen	0-4ml/24 hr.	↑Hemolytic jaundice (normal value in post-hepatic obstructive jaundice)
Urine bilirubin	None	↑Post-hepatic obstructive jaundice (none in hemolytic jaundice)

Table 18-7. *Blood Gases*

Arterial Blood Gases	Normal Values
pH	7.35-7.45
pO_2	80-100mmHg
O_2 saturation	95-100%
pCO_2	35-45mmHg
HCO_3-	22-26mmEq/1 (is also reflected in CO_2 content in electrolyte results)

BLOOD GAS ABNORMALITIES

7.35-7.45 pH	35-45mmHg pCO_2	22-26mEq HCO_3-	Assessment
↓	↑	normal	Respiratory Acidosis
↑	↓	normal	Respiratory Alkalosis
↓	normal	↓	Metabolic Acidosis
↑	normal	↑	Metabolic Alkalosis
↓	↑	↓	Mixed Resp. & Metabolic Acidosis
↑	↓	↑	Mixed Resp. & Metabolic Alkalosis
↓normal	↑	↑	Compensated Respiratory Acidosis
↑normal	↓	↓	Compensated Respiratory Alkalosis
↓normal	↓	↓	Compensated Metabolic Acidosis
↑normal	↑	↑	Compensated Metabolic Alkalosis

Table 18-8.   Coagulation Time

Coagulation Tests	Normal values
Bleeding time (Ivy)	1-5 min.
(Duke)	1-3 min.
Clotting time (Lee-White)	7-15 min.
Prothrombin time	12-14 sec.
(to be compared with control)	
Activated partial thromboplastin time (PTT)	35-40 sec.

Anticoagulation Drugs

Heparin	**Coumadin**
Anticoagulant drug interferes with thrombin formation	Interferes with liver absorption, synthesis and storage of Vitamin K.
Peak 20-30 min. Duration 4 hours	Depresses factors II, VII, IX, X.
Anticoagulant therapy levels 2-2½ times normal blood values	Onset 10 hours Peak 2-5 days Duration 10-14 days
Continuous IV. PTT 60-100 sec. q 6 hrs. 55-75 sec.	Anticoagulant therapeutic levels 1½-2½ times control of Protime 20-30 seconds
Coagulation time 30-45 min. (Lee-White)	

166

COAGULATION PATHWAY

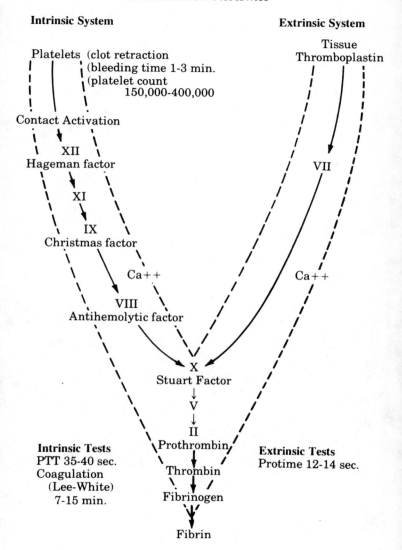

Intrinsic System

Platelets (clot retraction
(bleeding time 1-3 min.
(platelet count
150,000-400,000

Contact Activation

XII
Hageman factor

XI

IX
Christmas factor

Ca^{++}

VIII
Antihemolytic factor

Extrinsic System

Tissue
Thromboplastin

VII

Ca^{++}

X
Stuart Factor

V

II
Prothrombin

Thrombin

Fibrinogen

Fibrin

Intrinsic Tests
PTT 35-40 sec.
Coagulation
(Lee-White)
7-15 min.

Extrinsic Tests
Protime 12-14 sec.

References
Davidsohn I, and Henry, JB; (Eds.): *Todd-Sanford's Clinical Diagnosis by Laboratory Methods* (15th ed.). Philadelphia: W. B. Saunders Co., 1974

Holstead JA: *The Laboratory in Clinical Medicine: Interpretation and Adaptation.* Philadelphia: W. B. Saunders Co., 1976

Shrake, K: "The ABC's of ABG's." *Nursing 79,* September, p. 26-33, 1979

SELECTED CARDIAC FINDINGS

Table 19-1.   EKG Configurations

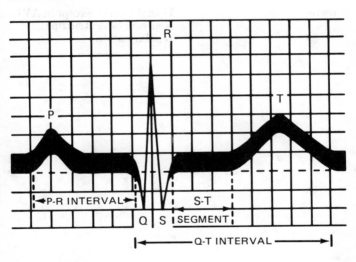

Electrical pattern of cardiac cycle.

p wave   < .10 sec.
                                Best seen in Lead II
                                Represents atrial
                                depolarization

PR interval	.12-.20 sec. Shows conduction through AV node, bundle of His, bundle branches
QRS complex	.06-.10 Represents ventricular depolarization
ST segment	Normally at isoelectric line
QT interval	.36-.44 sec. Represents ventricular systole, depolarization and repolarization of ventricles
T wave	Upright curve except in AVR Represents ventricular repolarization

Table 19-2. EKG Abnormalities in Myocardial Infarction

EKG Pattern	Figure
Normal EKG pattern (A)	
Ischemia—Depressed or inverted T wave (B)	

Injury—ST segment elevation or depression (C)

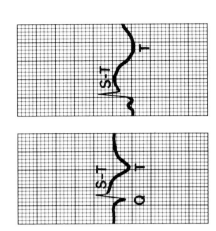

Necrosis—Q wave (D)
To be considered pathological Q waves must be:
  New Finding
  Duration .04 sec. or longer
  Usually 4m or greater in height
  Appear in leads that do not usually have Q waves

Table 19-3. EKG Interpretation of Myocardial Infarction

Leads	Inferior MI	Anterior MI	Septal MI	Lateral MI	Posterior MI
I				⋎	
II	⋎ ⋎				
III					
AVR					
AVL				⋎	
AVF	⋎				
V1	Normal ⋎	⋎	⋎		Tall R, ST depression, tall, upright T waves
V2	Normal ⋎ in children and blacks	⋎	⋎		
V3		⋎	⋎		
V4		⋎ ⋎			Tall R, ST depression, tall upright T waves
V5				⋎ ⋎	
V6					

173

Isoenzymes for Myocardial Infarction. An isoenzyme is a varied molecular form of a particular enzyme. For example, enzymes which indicate tissue damage can be analyzed by their particular isoenzyme which will then indicate the particular tissue of the body which has been damaged. In acute myocardial infarctions, the isoenzymes of lactic dehydrogenase (LDH) and creatine phosphokinase (CPK) are most frequently used to determine the presence of an infarction.

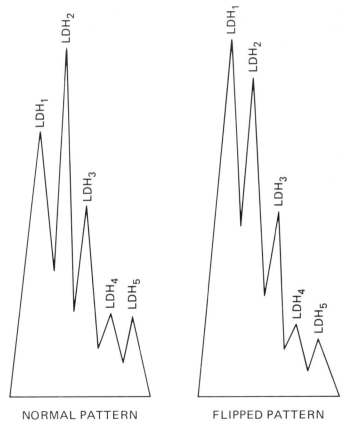

NORMAL PATTERN   FLIPPED PATTERN

Figure 19-1. Profile of the "Flipped LDH"

Lactic Dehydrogenase. If there has been an acute myocardial infarction, the LDH assumes the flipped profile usually 12 to 24 hours after the acute episode. This flipped pattern is also seen in acute renal infarction, and in hemolysis associated with prosthetic heart valves, hemolytic anemia, and pernicious anemia. However, the LDH flipped pattern with the proper clinical picture is usually diagnostic of an acute myocardial infarction.

Creatine Phosphatase. There are three CPK isoenzymes. The presence of CPK's usually indicates damaged myocardium. Following an acute myocardial infarction CPK_2 appears four to eight hours after chest pain, reaches peak activity at 18 to 24 hours.

CPK_2 is also found in the serum of patients with certain neuromuscular disorders, and other cardiac disorders.

Summary. In a patient with the proper clinical picture, the presence of CPK_2 in the serum followed by the LDH flipped pattern is nearly 100% predictive of an acute myocardial infarction.

REFERENCE
Galen RS: *Diagnosis.* March/April, 36-42, 1979

Axis Deviation. The orientation of the heart's electrical activity in the frontal plane is termed "axis." The axis can be determined from any two limb leads. Using limb leads I and aVF and looking at the positive (+) or negative (−) deflection of the QRS complex, you can place the axis in its appropriate quadrant. See Fig. 19-2 for quick reference.

A more precise location of axis can be achieved by comparing the size of the QRS complexes in the two leads, plotting them on the axis chart and drawing a horizontal line through the aVF point and a vertical line through the Lead I point. Where the two lines intersect will be the electrical axis.

Axis Deviation

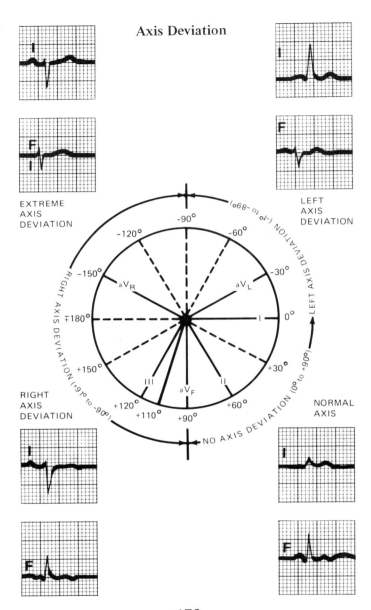

EXTREME AXIS DEVIATION

LEFT AXIS DEVIATION

RIGHT AXIS DEVIATION

NORMAL AXIS

LEFT AXIS DEVIATION (-1° to -89°)

RIGHT AXIS DEVIATION (+91° to -90°)

NO AXIS DEVIATION (0° to +90°)

REFERENCES

Andreoli K, Fawkes VH, Zipes D, et al.: *Comprehensive cardiac care* (4th ed.). St. Louis: C. V. Mosby, 1979

Bates, B: *Guide to physical examination* (2nd ed.). Philadelphia: J. B. Lippincott, 1979

Beeson PB, and McDermott W: *Textbook of medicine* (14th ed.). Philadelphia: W. B. Saunders, 1975

Carini, E and Owens G: *Neurological and neurosurgical nursing* (5th ed.). St. Louis: C. V. Mosby, 1970

DeGowin E and DeGowin R: *Bedside diagnostic examination.* New York: Macmillan, 1976

Davidsohn I. and J.B. Henry (Eds.) *Todd-Sanford's clinical diagnosis by laboratory methods* (15th ed.). Philadelphia: W. B. Saunders, 1974.

Galen RS: *Diagnosis,* March/April, 1979

Gilles DA, and Alyn I: *Patient assessment and management by the nurse practitioner.* Philadelphia: W. B. Saunders, 1974

Harvey AM, Johns RJ, Owens AH, et al.: *The principles and practice of medicine* (19th ed.). New York: Appleton-Century-Crofts, 1976

Holstead JA: *The laboratory in clinical medicine: interpretation and adaptation.* Philadelphia: W. B. Saunders Co., 1976

Malasanos L, Barkoukas V, Moss M, et al.: *Health assessment.* St. Louis: C. V. Mosby, 1977

McClintic JR: *Basic anatomy and physiology of the human body.* New York: John Wiley and Sons, 1975

Sauve, MJ and Pecheru A: *Concepts and skills in physical assessment.* Philadelphia: W. B. Saunders, 1977

Sherman, J and Fields S: *Guide to patient evaluation* (3rd ed.). Flushing, New York: Medical Examination Publishing, 1978

Shrake K: "The ABC's of ABG's." *Nursing 79,* September, 1979

Tilkian AG and Conover MB: *Understanding heart sounds and murmurs.* Philadelphia: W. B. Saunders, 1979

Vaughan-Wrobel B, and Henderson B: *The problem oriented system in nursing—a workbook.* St. Louis: C. V. Mosby, 1976

Widmann, FK: *Goodale's clinical interpretation of laboratory tests* (7th ed.). Philadelphia: F. A. Davis, 1973

INDEX

182